The Regulation of Medical Care: Is The Price Too High?

6-4

The Regulation of Medical Care: Is The Price Too High?

John C. Goodman

Cato Public Policy Research Monograph No. 3

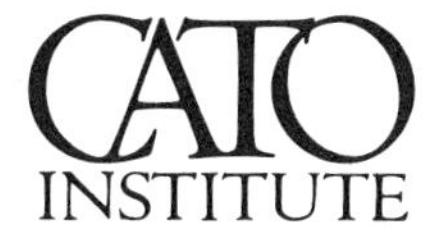

Library of Congress Cataloging in Publication Data

Goodman, John C
The regulation of medical care.

(Cato public policy research monograph; no. 3)
Includes bibliographical references.
1. Medical policy—United States. 2. Medical economics—United States. 3. Competition—United States. 4. Medical laws and legislation—United States. I. Title. II. Series: Cato Institute.
Cato public policy research monograph; no. 3.
RA395.A3G66 362.1'068 80-25397
ISBN 0-932790-23-2

Printed in the United States of America.

CATO INSTITUTE
747 Front Street
San Francisco, California 94111

CONTENTS

The author would like to acknowledge gratefully the assistance in the preparation of the manuscript of Susan M. Tully, Bridgett T. Gaines, Rosemary Curran, and Sue Stevens.

I. INTRODUCTION

> *My thesis is that a congeries of legislatively and professionally conceived and executed trade restraints have heretofore prevented the market from functioning with close to its potential effectiveness and that restoration of a market regime offers the best hope for solving the nation's health care problem in all of its dimensions.*
>
> Clark C. Havighurst
> "HMOs and the Market
> for Health Services"

That there is a crisis in the American health care system seems to be widely acknowledged. Within the last year *Time* and *Newsweek* magazines devoted cover stories to the so-called crisis, and ABC "World Nightly News" spent five straight nights exploring its various dimensions.

Much of what is considered a "crisis" in our health care system is not really a crisis at all. The fact that we are spending more of our national income on health care than ever before is hardly surprising. It is natural and inevitable that as we become more wealthy, we will want to spend more of our income on health care. This is a historical phenomenon that has been observed in all countries over time. Nor is it surprising that what we casually refer to as "health care" is becoming more expensive. New innovations and inventions in medical science have expanded the range of services that doctors and hospitals can offer, and the real cost of this new technology is frequently quite high. But the advent of new medical technology can hardly be described as a "crisis." These developments in no way make us worse off. They do not destroy old options, they merely create new ones.

Nonetheless there is a genuine crisis, or at least a major problem, in the health care marketplace. The problem is that we do not get our money's worth for the dollars we spend on health care. Under a different set of institutions, we could get more health care for the dollars we are now spending; or, put alternatively, we could obtain the same quantity and quality of health care we now receive at a lower cost.

Why does this problem exist? Most public discussions of the issue imply that the failures of our health care system are failures inherent in a free market for medical care. Such a conclusion inevitably points in the direction of an age-old "solution": more government regulation.

The thesis of this book is quite different: Most of the problems we encounter in the market for health care arise not because the free market has failed but because it has not yet been tried.

As the reader will soon discover, I place much, but not all, of the blame for this state of affairs squarely at the feet of organized medicine, which has, for over 100 years, sought and obtained special privileges from government. These special privileges take the form of restrictions on free competition in the marketplace. Although organized medicine's long and extensive involvement with government deserves much of the blame for the current state of affairs, this book should not be taken as an indictment of the medical profession itself. On the contrary, there are a great many medical practitioners today who would gladly trade their status as regulated professionals for the opportunity to freely compete in an unhampered health care market.

II. CONTROLS ON WHO MAY PRACTICE: THE PHYSICIAN

> *"First, . . . [the clockmaker's] art is not only by the bad workmanship of strangers disgraced, but [the clockmakers are] dis-enabled to make sale of their commodities at such rates as they may reasonably live by.*
>
> *"Secondly, for that divers strangers inhabiting in and about London do usually go to gentlemen's and noblemen's chambers and other places to offer their works to sale, which (for the most part) being not serviceable (the parties buying the same for the outward show only, which commonly is beautiful), are much deceived in the true value, which rests in the in-work only, and cannot be amended or by the buyers perceived.*
>
> *"Thirdly, . . . through the buyer's unskilfulness and the fugitiveness of the sellers, divers persons of worth have been utterly deceived of their money by strangers under colour of fair words and promises.*
>
> *"Fourthly, . . . said strangers . . . grow so bold to intrude upon the privileges of this kingdom, that is not only to take apprentices with money for few years, but also to keep open shop, and those apprentices never being able to be made good workmen by them, the said strangers . . . leave those apprentices to make most unserviceable work, whereby the said art is not only disgraced but the buyers much abused and deceived."*
>
> Petition by the London Clockmakers, 1622

In 1958 Professor Reuben Kessel wrote a trailblazing article, "Price Discrimination in Medicine,"[1] arguing that the American Medical Association (AMA) acts as a cartel agent for the country's physicians. All of the AMA's major policies, Kessel maintained, are designed to promote a single objective: to increase to the maximum the incomes of

[1]Reuben A. Kessel, "Price Discrimination in Medicine," *Journal of Law and Economics* 1 (October 1958): 20–53. Kessel was not the first to contend that the AMA runs a cartel for its members, but he was the first to rationalize all of the major AMA policies in terms of cartel objectives.

its members. Kessel carefully examined a large number of AMA policies, finding them consistent with his thesis and inconsistent with the publicly stated aims of the AMA.

How is it possible for an organization to run successfully a cartel consisting of more than 300,000 doctors? After all, economists can find few historical instances of successful cartels, even when collusion required the cooperation of only a handful of participants. Kessel's answer is that the AMA derived its monopoly power from the state: Like the clockmakers of seventeenth-century England, the leaders of organized medicine sought and obtained favorable legal restrictions on the entrance to, and conditions of, medical practice.

Early History

A genuinely free market in medical care did not emerge until the middle of the nineteenth century.[2] Between 1830 and 1850 many of the medical licensing laws that remained as legacies of the colonial period and the earliest years of the republic were repealed.[3] Ronald Hamowy has described the condition of the American medical profession at the close of the Civil War:

> The profession was, throughout the country, unlicensed, and anyone who had the inclination to set himself up as a physician could do so, the exigencies of the market alone determining who would prove successful in the field and who would not. Medical schools abounded, the great bulk of which were privately owned and operated, and the prospective student could gain admission to even the best of them without great difficulty. With free entry into the profession possible and education in medicine cheap and readily available, large numbers of men entered practice.[4]

The AMA was established as a permanent national organization at Philadelphia in 1847, and in a short time it became the spokesman for

[2]This section is largely based on the excellent treatment of the subject in Ronald Hamowy, "The Early Development of Medical Licensing Laws in the United States, 1875–1900," *Journal of Libertarian Studies* 3, no. 1 (1979): 73–119.

[3]Although twenty states and the District of Columbia had some form of licensing prior to 1850, these laws were commonly short-lived and poorly enforced. Five states provided no penalty for practicing without a license, and in six more the penalty, at worst, was that unlicensed practitioners could not sue for recovery of fees. Only in New York, South Carolina, Georgia, and Louisiana did unlicensed practitioners face the possibility of imprisonment. See Joseph F. Kett, *The Formation of the American Medical Association: The Role of Institutions, 1780–1860* (New Haven: Yale University Press, 1968), pp. 181–84; William G. Rothstein, *American Physicians in the Nineteenth Century: From Sect to Science* (Baltimore: Johns Hopkins University Press, 1972), pp. 332–39.

[4]Hamowy, p. 73.

practitioners of orthodox medicine in the United States. The AMA tirelessly stressed the noble goals of raising the quality of care for patients and protecting uninformed consumers from the activities of charlatans. Yet behind the avowed devotion to serve the public selflessly was the incessant, and often thinly disguised, concern with the financial well-being of the medical practitioner.

For example, a report submitted by the committee on educational standards to the Philadelphia meeting in 1847 was unusually candid. The following excerpt from the report suggests that the spirit of the London clockmaker's petition quoted at the head of this chapter was alive and thriving 200 years later in the minds of the committee members:

> The very large number of physicians in the United States . . . has frequently been the subject of remark. To relieve the diseases of something more than twenty millions of people, we have an army of Doctors amounting by a recent computation to forty thousand, which allows one to about every five hundred inhabitants. And if we add to the 40,000 the long list of irregular practitioners who swarm like locusts in every part of the country, the proportion of patients will be still further reduced. No wonder, then, that the profession of medicine has measurably ceased to occupy the elevated position which once it did; *no wonder that the merest pittance in the way of remuneration is scantily doled out even to the most industrious in our ranks* — and no wonder that the intention, at one time correct and honest, will occasionally succumb to the cravings of hard necessity.[5]

It is ironic that most of the practitioners of unorthodox ("irregular") medicine at the time were probably of greater benefit — or, at least, of less harm — to their patients than the practitioners of orthodoxy.[6] A second irony is that the committee on medical education proceeded to

[5]"Proceedings of the National Medical Convention held in the City of Philadelphia, in May, 1847," *The New York Journal of Medicine* 9 (July 1847): 115. Emphasis added.

[6]According to Hamowy, regular medicine in the nineteenth century relied heavily on treatment consisting of "bloodletting, blistering, and the administration of massive doses of compounds of mercury, antinomy, and other mineral poisons as purgatives and emetics, followed by arsenical compounds thought to act as tonics." The two major schools of nonorthodox medicine were electicism and homeopathy. The former relied exclusively on botanical remedies, steam baths, and rest. The latter advocated small doses of drugs, which, when tested in a healthy person, produced symptoms most closely approximating the symptomology of the disease. Homeopathic doctors were also strong proponents of fresh air, sunshine, bed rest, proper diet, and personal hygiene — therapeutic remedies that the practitioners of regular medicine regarded as of little or no value. See Hamowy, pp. 73–74.

recommend educational standards so high that it is doubtful that more than a handful of the delegates to the AMA convention had themselves satisfied the requirements. Indeed, one historian has concluded that "rigid enforcement of the AMA's preliminary standards would have closed down practically every medical school in the country and would have depleted the ranks of formally educated physicians in a few years."[7]

Following an exhaustive study of the early development of medical licensing laws in the United States, Hamowy has concluded that the goals of orthodox practitioners in general, and of the AMA in particular, were threefold: (1) to establish medical licensing laws that would restrict entry into the profession and thus secure a more stable (and lucrative) financial climate for physicians than had existed under uninhibited competition; (2) to destroy the proprietary (for profit) medical schools and replace them with a few nonprofit institutions that would provide extensive, thorough training in medicine, with a longer required period of study and a smaller and more select student body; and (3) to eliminate heterodox medical sects, generally seen as unwelcome competitive forces within the profession.[8]

Hamowy points out that in attempting to achieve these objectives, AMA spokesmen displayed a "selfless concern for the welfare of a befuddled and helpless public, preyed upon by incompetents and purveyors of poisons."[9] Yet every law designed to restrict the practice of medicine was enacted not on the crest of widespread public demand, but rather "largely because of intense pressure from the medical profession" itself.[10]

But how much concern did the leadership of organized medicine really have for the victims of "incompetents and purveyors of poisons?" Consider the fact that the AMA steadfastly supported grandfather clauses in every licensing law it proposed: These clauses exempted existing practitioners from the requirements of the laws, and burdened only those *entering* the profession. In fact, when Minnesota enacted a medical practice act in 1887 that required that "all persons hereafter commencing the practice of medicine and surgery" in Minnesota "present evidence of attendance on three courses of lectures of six months each" in a medical school, the *Journal of the American*

7Rothstein, p. 120.

8Hamowy, p. 75.

9Ibid., p. 90.

10Ibid., p. 96.

Medical Association complained bitterly that the law might be interpreted to apply to established practitioners coming to Minnesota from other states as well as to those just entering the profession.[11] It is also noteworthy that licensing laws supported by the AMA left physicians free to practice medicine according to any system of therapeutics they chose once they had obtained a license to practice.[12]

Consider also the grounds for the refusal to grant or revocation of a license included in AMA-sponsored legislation. By 1907 forty-two states and territories had such provisions. The most common causes for refusal or revocation were "dishonorable" or "unprofessional" conduct. In most instances these terms were interpreted to mean a violation of the AMA's code of ethics. Yet in only two states — Iowa and South Dakota — was incompetence a grounds for revocation of a certificate to practice.[13]

In 1888 the *Journal of the American Medical Association* editorialized that "*Wholesome* competition is the life of trade; unrestricted competition may be the death of it. . . . Wholesome competition is the life of *trade*; but competition does not make or increase the business of the physician."[14] That the AMA was far more concerned with competition than with the welfare of the public is abundantly clear from the historical record. In 1898 the New York State medical fraternity proposed a statute that would have prevented free vaccination and the administration of free diphtheria antitoxin on the grounds that the practice was "inimic to the best [financial] welfare of young medical men."[15] The AMA's code of medical ethics included an injunction against administering to affluent patients without compensation. Such

[11]See "Medical Legislation," *Journal of the American Medical Association* 10 (28 January 1888): 113–14.

[12]See "The License to Practice," *Journal of the American Medical Association* 12 (25 May 1889): 741. For a summary of court rulings (which generally supported the AMA position) on this issue, see Harold Wright Holt, "The Need for Administrative Discretion in the Regulation of the Practice of Medicine," *Cornell Law Quarterly* 16 (June 1931): 508.

[13]Hamowy, pp. 106–7, n. 32. For a synopsis of the revocation provisions in the various medical practice acts as of 1907, see "Medical Practice Laws," *American Medical Association Bulletin* 3 (15 November 1907): 80–87.

[14]"Competition, Supply and Demand, and Medical Education," *Journal of the American Medical Association* 11 (15 September 1888): 382–83.

[15]See "Proposed 'Practical' Medical Legislation for New York State," *Journal of the American Medical Association* 30 (12 March 1898): 625.

administrations were deemed "dishonorable" and "unprofessional" because they tended to injure other physicians financially.[16]

In addition, organized medicine vigorously sought to eliminate competition from any unlicensed person who would treat the sick for compensation, regardless of the form of treatment and its effect on the patient. For example, in most states physicians were successful in broadening the definition of medical practice to include drugless and spiritual healers (e.g., Christian Scientists, osteopaths, and chiropractors).[17] At the urging of organized medicine, courts ruled that it was not a defense that patients knowingly accepted the mode of treatment offered, nor that patients may have benefited by the treatment![18]

In one interesting case, the Nebraska Supreme Court in 1894 ruled that a Christian Science practitioner had violated the state's medical practice act by accepting compensation in return for treating solely by prayer those who called on him.[19] A similar decision was reached by the Ohio Supreme Court in 1905. In that case it was ruled that Christian Science treatment in return for a fee constituted the practice of medicine, even though the cure was to come from God and not from the defendant.[20]

By 1901 all states and territories (except Alaska and Oklahoma) had instituted medical examining boards. Of the fifty-one jurisdictions, thirty required candidates for a license to undergo an examination and to present a diploma in medicine; seven required either an examination or a diploma; and two made the M.D. degree a prerequisite for the practice of medicine. Despite these regulations, the absolute number of physicians continued to increase — from 82,000 in 1880 to

16Chapter II, article 5, section 9 of the code of medical ethics, adopted at the first AMA convention read: "A wealthy physician should not give advice *gratis* to the affluent because it is an injury to his professional brethren. The office of physician can never be supported as an exclusively beneficent one; and it is defrauding in some degree, the common funds for its support, when fees are dispensed with, which might justly be claimed." See "Code of Medical Ethics," *The New York Journal of Medicine* 9 (September 1847). The injunction apparently does not apply to ministering *gratis* to another physician — a practice that is quite widespread. See the analysis of the practice in Reuben A. Kessel, "Price Discrimination in Medicine," pp. 20–53.

17Hamowy, p. 96.

18Ibid., p. 98. For an account of the rise of medical licensing laws in terms of their reception by the courts, see Lawrence M. Friedman, "Freedom of Contract and Occupational Licensing, 1890–1910: A Legal and Social Study," *California Law Review* 53 (1965): 487–534.

19*State* v. *Buswell*, 40 Nebraska 158, 58 N.W. 728 (1894).

20*State* v. *Marble*, 72 Ohio State 21, 73 N.E. 1063 (1905).

120,000 in 1900. The number of physicians per 100,000 population fell, however, from 163 in 1880 to 157 by the turn of the century.[21]

Nonetheless, in 1901 the *Journal of the American Medical Association* continued to complain about overcrowded conditions in the medical professions.[22] Hamowy explains why:

> Licensing laws mandating an examination were clearly not sufficiently restrictive to severely limit the numbers of new physicians entering the profession, even when these laws also required a diploma in medicine. The answer was to lie in statutes which both required a diploma and, in addition, empowered the state examining boards to exclude graduates of "sub-standard" colleges from consideration for licensure.[23]

The Flexner Report

During the colonial period, medical education, like the education for most other learned occupations, was obtained by apprenticeship. Young men desiring to enter the medical profession would indenture themselves to a practicing physician in return for the training received. However, formal classroom training began gradually to supplement the training received at the master's side and eventually to replace it.

As noted above, during the latter part of the nineteenth century medical schools (many of them proprietary) were flourishing. In 1870 there were approximately 75 medical schools in the United States. This number grew to 100 by 1880, to 133 by 1890, and to 160 by the turn of the century.[24] Between 1900 and 1907, over five thousand graduates a year were being absorbed into the medical profession, despite the licensing laws designed to stem the tide of new entrants.[25]

In 1906 the Council on Medical Education of the AMA undertook an inspection of existing medical schools and found the training fully acceptable in only eighty-two of them. The results of this report were never published, however, because the council decided that its report would receive more widespread public acceptance if it were released

21Hamowy, p. 102.

22Ibid., p. 103. See "Oversupply of Medical Graduates," *Journal of the American Medical Association* 37 (27 July 1901): 270.

23Hamowy, p. 103.

24See U.S. Department of Health, Education and Welfare, U.S. Public Health Service, *Health Manpower Source Book*, section 9, "Physicians, Dentists and Professional Nurses" (1959), p. 9.

25Hamowy, p. 103.

under the auspices of the highly respected Carnegie Foundation for the Advancement of Teaching. As Arthur Bevan, head of the Council on Medical Education, explained, "If we could obtain the publication and approval of our work by the Carnegie Foundation . . . it would assist materially in securing the results we are attempting to bring about."[26]

The AMA's efforts were successful. In 1910 the Carnegie Foundation commissioned Abraham Flexner to perform what amounted to a repetition of the AMA's inspection and grading of medical schools. Flexner lacked the qualifications to perform the task for which he was commissioned: He was not a physician; he was not a scientist; he was never a medical educator. He had an undergraduate degree in arts and was the owner and operator of a for-profit preparatory school in Louisville, Kentucky.[27]

Flexner's method of evaluating existing medical schools consisted of conducting a grand inspection tour — nothing more, nothing less. Sometimes he evaluated an entire school in one afternoon. His method for measuring the qualifications of a medical school was to compare it to the medical school at Johns Hopkins. He was accompanied on the tour by the secretary of the AMA's Council on Medical Education, N. P. Colwell, who provided him with the results of the AMA's previous labors. Flexner apparently accepted ample assistance from the AMA and spent many hours at its Chicago headquarters working on the preparation of his report.[28]

The picture Flexner painted of those schools deemed unacceptable is noteworthy:

> These enterprises — for the most part they can be called schools or institutions only by courtesy — were frequently set up regardless of opportunity or need: in small towns as readily as in large, and at times almost in the heart of the wilderness. . . . Wherever and whenever the roster of untitled practitioners rose above half a dozen, a medical school was likely at any moment to be precipitated. Nothing was really essential but professors. . . . Little or no investment was therefore involved. A hall could be cheaply rented and rude benches were inexpensive. Janitor service was unknown and is even now relatively rare. Occasional dissections in time supplied a skeleton — in whole or in part — and a box of odd bones. Other equipment there was practically none. The teaching was, except for a little

[26]Arthur Bevan, "Cooperation in Medical Education and Medical Service," *Journal of the American Medical Association* 90 (1928): 1175.

[27]Reuben A. Kessel, "The AMA and the Supply of Physicians," *Law and Contemporary Problems* (Spring 1970): 269.

[28]Ibid., pp. 268–69.

> anatomy, wholly didactic. The schools were essentially private ventures, money-making in spirit and object.... Income was simply divided among the lecturers, who reaped a rich harvest, besides, through the consultations which the loyalty of their former students threw in their hands.... No applicant for instruction who could pay his fees or sign his note was turned down.... The examinations, brief, oral, and secret, plucked almost none at all....[29]

A school-by-school review of Flexner's report confirms this overall assessment. Yet it is difficult to agree with Flexner's conclusion that the country might have been "spared [this] demoralizing experience in medical education...."[30] For one thing, Flexner made a serious error in economic reasoning. He was examining the *inputs* of these schools, not the *outputs*. Instead of finding out how qualified the graduates of these particular schools were, he looked at how they were taught, which is like assigning grades on the basis of how many hours a student spends studying for an exam rather than on the basis of his actual performance on the exam. (It is interesting that Flexner's brother, who became a very distinguished physician, graduated from one of the schools put out of business as a result of the Flexner Report.)[31]

As Kessel has pointed out, Flexner also mistakenly applied Gresham's law to the market for physicians' services.[32] Flexner argued that through the operation of Gresham's law, poor quality physicians drove out of the market the services of those with higher qualifications. Not only is Gresham's law inapplicable, but there is little evidence of the effect that Flexner claimed to have observed.[33] In addition, Flexner failed to realize that raising the standards of medical education is not necessarily in the public interest. Higher standards imply higher costs of medical care. As Kessel notes, "[Flexner's] argument is on a par

[29]Abraham Flexner, *Medical Education in the United States and Canada*, Bulletin No. 4, The Carnegie Foundation for the Advancement of Teaching (Boston: D. B. Updike, The Merrymount Press, 1910), pp. 6–7.

[30]Ibid., p. 6.

[31]Kessel, "The AMA and the Supply of Physicians," p. 269, n. 6.

[32]Kessel, "Price Discrimination in Medicine," p. 27.

[33]Gresham's law states that bad money drives out good. It is applicable, however, only in the presence of legal tender laws — where sellers and creditors are forbidden by law to refuse all forms of specie deemed "legal tender." Naturally, if buyers and debtors have a choice they would rather make payment with the least valuable form of specie. In the absence of legal tender laws, however, sellers and creditors are not obligated to accept any particular form of payment. Under these circumstances Gresham's law tends to work in reverse: "Good money drives out bad." See Murray Rothbard, *What Has Government Done to Our Money?* (Colorado Springs, Colo.: Pine Tree Press, 1963).

with arguing that we should keep all cars of a quality below Cadillacs, Chryslers, and Lincolns off the market."[34]

On the whole, the public was not necessarily ill-served by the existing institutions of medical education. After all, this was a period when

> the United States was growing both in numbers and in size at a virtually frantic pace. Great frontiers were being opened and settled which required [an] increased number of individuals with medical training.... The fact remains ... that students remained eager to enroll in such schools and were quite willing to pay fees to receive the training offered. Investment in such training seems to have been profitable.[35]

Presumably it was profitable because the training led to services for which people were willing to pay.

The Flexner Report had an enormous impact on medical education in this country. Indeed, Kessel has written that "If impact on public policy is the criterion of importance, the Flexner Report must be regarded as one of the most important reports ever written."[36] Legislators were convinced by the report that only graduates of first class (class A) medical schools ought to be licensed. The classification of institutions was either explicitly or implicitly delegated to the AMA. In time, every state established standards of acceptability for licensing doctors. These standards were set either by statute or by formal and informal rules of state medical examining boards, provided that the boards consider only the graduates of schools approved by the AMA or the American Association of Medical Colleges.[37]

Ultimately the Flexner Report led to the large-scale closing of those medical schools that failed to meet the high educational standards established by the AMA.[38] By exercising its power to certify, the

[34]Kessel, "Price Discrimination in Medicine," p. 27, n. 18.

[35]Cotton M. Lindsay and James M. Buchanan, "The Organization and Financing of Medical Care in the United States," in *Health Services Financing* (London: British Medical Association, 1974), pp. 540–41.

[36]Kessel, "Price Discrimination in Medicine," p. 28.

[37]David R. Hyde, Payson Wolff, Anne Gross, and Elliott Lee Hoffman, "The American Medical Association: Power, Purpose and Politics in Organized Medicine," *Yale Law Journal* 65 (May 1954): 969.

[38]It is interesting that Flexner's standards appear to have been higher than the AMA's standards. Whereas the initial AMA study rated eighty-two schools as class A in 1906, Flexner rated only seventy-two schools that high in 1910. See Kessel, "The AMA and the Supply of Physicians," p. 269, n. 8.

TABLE 2.1

Medical Schools: 1850 to 1970[1] [2]

Year	Number	Students	Graduates
1850	52	—	—
1860	65	—	—
1870	75	—	—
1880	100	11,826	3,241
1890	133	15,404	4,454
1900	160	25,171	5,214
1910	131	21,526	4,440
1920	85	13,798	3,047
1930	76	21,597	4,565
1940	77	21,271	5,097
1950	79	25,103	5,553
1960	91	31,999	7,508
1970	107	39,666	8,799

SOURCE: U.S. Bureau of the Census, *Historical Statistics of the United States, Colonial Times to 1970, Bicentennial Edition, Part 2* (Washington, D.C., 1975), Series B 275–290, pp. 75–76.

[1]Figures are for academic session ending in specified years.

[2]Beginning 1954, includes Puerto Rico; beginning 1960, includes osteopaths and their schools.

AMA reduced the number of medical schools in the United States from 131 in 1910 to 85 in 1920, 76 in 1930, and 69 in 1944.[39] (See table 2.1.) As a consequence, the number of medical students dropped dramatically. Whereas 21,526 students were attending medical school in 1910, the number declined to 13,798 by 1920 and did not again reach the 1910 figure until the 1940s.[40] (See table 2.2.) This decline did much to eliminate the "oversupply" of doctors that had so worried the editorialists at the *Journal of the American Medical Association.* Following the release of the Flexner Report, the ratio of doctors to population fell steadily over the next two decades. To see how effective the AMA's policies actually were, consider the fact that a doctor in 1963 had a far greater capability of helping his patients than a doctor did at the turn of the century, and, as a consequence, doctors in 1963 were in far greater demand. Yet the number of doctors per 100,000 population that year (146) was precisely what it was in the year the Flexner Report was written.[41]

[39]Kessel, "Price Discrimination in Medicine," p. 28.

[40]*Health Manpower Source Book,* section 9, p. 9.

[41]See Lindsay and Buchanan, table 2, p. 540.

TABLE 2.2

Physicians in the United States: 1850 to 1970

Year	Number[1]	Rates per 100,000 Population	Population per Physician
1850	40,755	176	568
1860	55,055	175	571
1870	60,000	150	667
1880	82,000	163	613
1890	100,180	159	629
1900	119,749	157	637
1910	135,000	146	685
1920	144,977[2]	137	729
1930	153,803[2]	125	800
1940	175,163	133	752
1950	203,400	134	746
1960	274,833	148	676
1970	348,328	166	602

SOURCE: U.S. Bureau of the Census, *Historical Statistics of the United States, Colonial Times to 1970, Bicentennial Edition, Part 2* (Washington, D.C., 1975), Series B 275–290, pp. 75–76.

[1]Beginning 1960, includes osteopaths.

[2]Census figures are used and may include physicians not in active medical practice.

The importance of the Flexner Report and the legislation that followed its publication cannot be overstated. Indeed, the effect of the report may be unique in American regulatory history. Professor Kessel explains why:

> The delegation by the state legislature to the AMA of the power to regulate the medical industry in the public interest is on a par with giving the American Iron and Steel Institute the power to determine the output of steel. This delegation of power by the states to the AMA, which was actively sought and solicited, placed this organization in a position of having to serve two masters who in part have conflicting interests. On the one hand, the AMA was given the task of providing an adequate supply of properly qualified doctors. On the other, the decision with respect to what is adequate training and an adequate number of doctors affects the pocketbooks of those who do the regulating as well as their closest business and personal associates. It is this power that has been given to the AMA that is the cornerstone of the monopoly power that has been imputed by economists to organized medicine.[42]

[42]Kessel, "Price Discrimination in Medicine," p. 29.

Subsequent AMA Policies Toward Medical Education

Kessel's contention that the AMA controls the supply of physicians has been disputed. For example, Mary Spahr writes of the "widespread but erroneous belief that the AMA governs the profession directly and determines who may practice medicine."[43] She argues that this power belongs to the state rather than to the AMA. Keith Leffler has written that

> [no] proponent of the view that the American Medical Association limits entry [into the profession] has documented how the American Medical Association directly influences the physician output of medical schools or how [the] American Medical Association successfully constrains new schools from opening. The criteria on which the Liaison Committee accredits medical schools are explicitly stated, publicly available, and infrequently changed. While the Liaison Committee has the power to impose inefficient training requirements, no implications about direct supply restrictions follow from that power.[44]

Leffler supports his position by pointing to two recent studies of medical schools. One, by Thomas Hall, created a model of medical schools that explained the variations over time in medical school capacity without any reference to the AMA's ability to restrict supply.[45] A second study, by Charles Hobbs, reported that in the legislative discussion of a proposal to construct an additional state-supported medical school in California, the possiblity that the AMA might withhold approval of the school was given no consideration.[46]

The power to license physicians and medical schools ultimately belongs to the state legislatures, but Kessel and others contend that this power has been delegated to the AMA by the state legislatures.[47]

[43]Mary Spahr, "Medicine's Neglected Control Lever," *Yale Review* 40 (Winter 1951): 25.

[44]Keith B. Leffler, *Explanation In Search of Facts: A Critique of "A Study of Physician's Fees"* (Coral Gables, Fla.: Law and Economics Center, University of Miami School of Law, 1978), p. 15. The Joint Liaison Committee on Medical Education was established in 1942 by the Council on Medical Education of the AMA. The committee consists of six representatives of the AMA, six representatives of the Association of American Medical Colleges, two public representatives, and one representative of the federal government. All states today have delegated the power to approve medical schools to this committee. See Edward H. Forgotson, Ruth Roemer, and Roger Newman, "Licensure of Physicians," *Washington University Law Quarterly*, 1967, p. 269.

[45]Thomas D. Hall, "The Behavior of Medical Schools as Nonprofit Firms" (Ph.D. diss., Department of Economics, University of California at Los Angeles, 1976).

[46]Charles E. Hobbs, *The Politics of Medical Education* (Los Angeles: Foundation for Research in Education and Economics, Medical Education Project, 1976).

[47]One of the early proponents of the view that the AMA has life and death powers over

Kessel admits this power need be of little concern to medical schools such as Johns Hopkins, for "it would be ludicrous not to classify this institution as a class A school."[48] Less distinguished schools, however, do have something to fear. And, despite Leffler's contention to the contrary, there are documented cases where the AMA has successfully threatened to exercise its power over these medical schools in order to bring about a reduction in the number of medical students being trained.

The most striking instance occurred during the Great Depression. Between 1929 and 1932 the incomes of physicians fell almost 40 percent.[49] The AMA responded to these hard times characteristically. In 1932 the report of a commission, largely financed by the AMA, complained of an "oversupply" of physicians and warned of "excessive economic competition," and "conditions in the profession which will not encourage students of superior ability and character to enter the profession."[50] The report concluded that "those responsible for medical education and for the licensing of physicians . . . should have the situation clearly before them."[51] That same year an editorial in the *Journal of the American Medical Association* echoed the charge of "oversupply,"[52] and two months later an article in the *JAMA* suggested that medical colleges be required "to reduce the number of graduates 25 percent each year until a ratio of 1 doctor to 2,000 of population is reached."[53] In 1933 the president of the AMA asserted that "there apparently is an overproduction of doctors,"[54] and the following year the new president of the AMA complained that "one is forced to the conviction that more doctors are being turned out than society needs and can comfortably reward."[55]

---

both medical schools and hospitals was Milton S. Mayer. See *Harper's* (December 1949), p. 27. The thesis has been expanded to book length by Elton Rayack. See his *Professional Power and American Medicine: The Economics of the American Medical Association* (Cleveland: World Publishing Co., 1967).

48Kessel, "Price Discrimination in Medicine," p. 29.

49U.S. Department of Commerce, *Survey of Current Business*, July 1951, p. 11.

50*Final Report of the Commission on Medical Education* (New York, 1932), p. 100.

51Ibid.

52*Journal of the American Medical Association* 99:1 (August 1932): 765.

53B. T. Beasley, "Economic Status of the Medical Profession — A Suggestion for Improvement," *Journal of the American Medical Association* 99:2 (October 1932): 1358.

54Dean Lewis: "The Place of the Clinic in Medical Practice," *Journal of the American Medical Association* 100:2 (June 1933): 1908.

55Walter Bierring, "The Family Doctor and the Changing Order," *Journal of the American Medical Association* 102:18–26 (June 1934): 1997.

What followed was a "little" Flexner Report. From 1934 to 1936 the AMA's Council on Medical Education surveyed eighty-nine medical schools in the United States and Canada. Not surprisingly, the council found that many schools had taken in larger numbers of students than they had been able to care for properly. However, after making contact with schools with errant admissions policies, the council reported that "most of the schools . . . which . . . allowed themselves to yield to the demands of this increasing number of applicants . . . have expressed their readiness to cooperate with us by reducing the size of their student body."[56]

The pressure exerted by the AMA on medical schools to cut back on enrollment had a substantial impact. Between the academic years 1933–34 and 1938–39 there was virtually no change in the number of applicants to medical schools in this country, yet that same period saw a decline of 17.9 percent in the number of acceptances. Seventy-four percent of this decline occurred within two years of the Council on Medical Education's 1935 warning to the medical schools against the admission of larger classes.[57]

A number of writers have observed that the AMA's changing positions on the proper standards for medical education correlate far more closely with the financial pressures faced by practicing physicians than with any clearly defined goals of medical training. For example, Kissam has written that

> the AMA's Council on Medical Education has been able to reduce the number of new physicians entering the profession by increasing the standards for accreditation of medical schools, thereby driving some schools out of business, discouraging new schools from opening, and reducing the size of others. . . . [yet the] quality standards imposed for physician licensure have never been carefully correlated with definitions of acceptable medical performance. . . . Most significantly, major "improvements" in standards for accredited medical schools generally have been imposed at times when physicians' incomes were relatively depressed and have been accompanied by open expressions of concern by leaders of organized medicine about the "over-crowded" medical profession.[58]

[56]Irvin D. Metzger, "The Federation of State Medical Boards," *Journal of the American Medical Association* 106:2 (April 1936): 1393; and Ray Lyman Wilbur, "Leadership in Medical Education," *Journal of the American Medical Association* 108:1 (March 1937): 771.

[57]Elton Rayack, "Restrictive Practices of Organized Medicine," *The Antitrust Bulletin* (1968), p. 675.

[58]Philip Kissam, "Physician's Assistant and Nurse Practitioner Laws: A Study of Health

There is some evidence, however, that in the postwar period control over the accreditation of medical schools has not been the major tool by which the AMA has sought to limit the supply of physicians.

Two consequences of the Flexner Report were the elimination of the proprietary medical schools and a growing gap between educational costs and tuition revenues for nonproprietary schools.[59] Higher accreditation standards meant more costly curriculum and laboratory requirements, which in turn meant that medical schools became increasingly reliant on external subsidies. As time went on, this reliance was directed more and more toward the federal government. As a consequence, the crucial determinant of how many doctors would be trained soon became the size of the available subsidies rather than the specific requirements of accreditation.

Elton Rayack has maintained that since World War II the AMA has been far more concerned with how many dollars flow through the federal money spigot to the nation's medical schools than with the educational standards maintained by those schools.[60] Having succeeded in making the schools dependent on external finances, the AMA proceeded to curtail the volume of subsidy.

For example, between 1946 and 1950 the AMA vigorously opposed all forms of federal aid to medical education that would have increased the supply of physicians. Between 1951 and 1958 the AMA reluctantly accepted the principle of one-time construction grants to medical schools — but only when there was a "demonstrated emergency." After 1958 the AMA conceded that federal assistance for construction purposes was necessary, but continued to oppose federal aid for scholarships and operational expenses. Only in recent years, with the rise of physicians' incomes, has the AMA relaxed its opposition to all forms of federal aid.

Like its positions on accreditation standards, the AMA's positions on the amount and proper form of federal subsidy appear to reflect primarily the financial concerns of practicing physicians. It is ludicrous to believe that the AMA's opposition to federal subsidies was

---

Law Reform," *Kansas Law Review* 24 (1975): 15. See also, Rosemary Stevens, *American Medicine and the Public Interest* (New Haven: Yale University Press, 1971) pp. 66–69; and Kessel, "The AMA and the Supply of Physicians," p. 282.

[59]Lee Benham, "Guilds and the Form of Competition in the Health Care Sector," in Warren Greenberg, ed., *Competition in the Health Care Sector: Past, Present and Future* (Germantown, Md.: Aspen Systems Corporation, 1978), p. 365.

[60]See Rayack, *Professional Power and American Medicine*, pp. 81–101.

based on some political principle. The organization's persistent struggle over the years to involve government in the health care market is well documented, and this activity has not been restricted to state legislatures. In 1900 the AMA launched a major effort to establish a federal department of health.[61] In the 1920s the *JAMA* editorially endorsed national health insurance, but the AMA withdrew this endorsement after evidence from several foreign countries with national health insurance systems suggested that under such systems doctors lose financially.[62]

In pursuit of its legislative goals the AMA has been willing to spare no expense. Between 1948 and 1968 the AMA spent more money on its Washington lobby than any other single pressure group, including the National Association of Manufacturers and the AFL–CIO.[63]

The Purpose of Licensing

After an extensive survey of the development of licensing laws in numerous professions, economist Thomas Moore concluded that "licensing raises the cost of entry, which, in turn, benefits practitioners already in the occupation at the time of licensing." Since benefiting practitioners is the principal effect of licensing, Moore concluded that it is also its principal purpose.[64] This view contrasts sharply, however, with the pronouncements of most regulatory authorities. A report issued by the Department of Health, Education and Welfare summarized the typical regulator's defense of licensing: "Theoretically," according to the report, the purpose of licensure is "to protect the public."[65]

What is the purpose of medical licensing? A careful look at the actual provisions of state licensing laws provides a revealing answer. The most recent survey of these provisions was conducted in 1967.[66] Since that time a number of modifications have been made by court rulings,

[61]Hamowy, pp. 93–94.

[62]A highly informative history of the AMA position on national health insurance is contained in Ronald Numbers, *Almost Persuaded: American Physicians and Compulsory Health Insurance, 1912–1920* (Baltimore: Johns Hopkins University Press, 1978).

[63]Rayack, "Restrictive Practices of Organized Medicine," p. 669.

[64]Thomas G. Moore, "The Purpose of Licensing," *Journal of Law and Economics* 4 (1961): 93–117.

[65]"Independent Practitioners Under Medicare, A Report to the Congress," Department of Health, Education and Welfare, 7, 1968.

[66]Forgotson, Roemer, and Newman, p. 253.

the actions of regulatory agencies, and by federal and state legislation, but the basic spirit of medical licensing laws today remains essentially as it was in 1967, or, for that matter, as it was at the turn of the century.

The most interesting aspect of state licensing laws, from the perspective of evaluating their purpose, is that a license is an *unlimited* license to perform all functions of health service.[67] A physician, once licensed, may theoretically perform all manner of surgery — including open heart surgery and brain surgery — even though the physician may never have received any special training as a surgeon. That licensed physicians may even provide dental service, even if they have received no training in dentistry is a remarkable feature of legislation whose alleged purpose is to assure the public that all those who offer to perform medical services have been adequately trained to do so.[68]

Another remarkable feature of state licensure laws is that a license constitutes a grant of lifetime tenure to the licensee. Medical licensure is

> lifetime licensure, without any legal requirement for updating qualifications or keeping abreast of new knowledge. Educational obsolescence becomes involved in the licensure process only when it is so egregious as to provide grounds for disciplinary action or revocation of license. It may be involved in the judicial process when it results in acts that are the subject of a malpractice suit.[69]

Although most states require licenses to be renewed periodically, license renewal is generally a routine clerical procedure requiring little more than the physician's signature and the payment of a nominal fee. No state requires the physician to show evidence of having updated his or her knowledge and credentials as a condition of maintaining a license in good standing.[70]

Reuben Kessel has asked why holders of automobile drivers' licenses are subject to reexamination and holders of licenses to practice medicine are not. Is medicine less important? Similarly, "why are commercial airline pilots subject to reexamination but not physicians?"[71] Clearly the

[67]Ibid.

[68]In 1967 two states, Texas and Georgia, specifically exempted physicians from the application of their dental practice acts, although such provisions appear to have been unnecessary. Ibid., n. 11.

[69]Ruth Roemer, "Licensing and Regulation of Medical and Medical-related Practitioners in Health Service Teams," *Medical Care* 9, no. 1 (1971): 47.

[70]Forgotson, Roemer, and Newman, p. 276.

[71]Kessel, "The AMA and the Supply of Physicians," p. 275.

answer has little to do with the welfare of patients. Kessel has also noted that in those rare instances where physicians *are* reexamined (for example, because a retired physician has allowed his license to lapse and wishes to resume practice), the examination he takes does not necessarily bear close resemblance to the examination taken by medical students.[72]

In 1967 the National Advisory Commission on Health Manpower recommended that relicensure of physicians be granted either on the basis of acceptable performance in continuing education programs or on the basis of examinations in the practitioner's specialty.[73] The medical profession has been singularly unenthusiastic about this recommendation, and no state has enacted these proposals.[74]

Not only are physicians not required to keep abreast with the state of medical science in their specialty in order to retain a license to practice, in some states a physician may continue to practice even if he is mentally ill. In 1967 only one state, Arizona, required that a candidate for a medical license be "physically and mentally able safely to engage in the practice of medicine."[75] Some statutes do establish mental illness or mental imcompetence as grounds for suspension or revocation of a license if the extent of the illness renders the physician "unsafe or unreliable as a practitioner." But other states permit a mentally ill physician to continue to practice, providing for license revocation or suspension only if the physician enters a mental hospital. Of course, while in a hospital the physician is unable to practice medicine in any event. Oregon provides for automatic suspension of a license in case of voluntary hospitalization exceeding twenty-five days, but allows other treatment without requiring proof of the "ability to practice medicine." The state of California provides for license suspension if the physician is voluntarily admitted or committed to a *state* hospital but has no such provision covering admissions to private hospitals.[76]

It may be argued that in those states where mental illness or mental incompetency is not listed as a specific ground for suspension or revocation of a license these conditions are covered by more general provisions proscribing any "conduct harmful to the public." For example a

[72]Ibid., p. 278.

[73]*Report of the National Advisory Commission on Health Manpower*, 1967, p. 40.

[74]Roemer, p. 47.

[75]Forgotson, Roemer, and Newman, p. 266.

[76]Ibid., p. 286.

provision is included in the Arizona statute that provides for suspension or revocation of a license for

> any conduct or practice contrary to recognized standards of ethics of the medical profession or any conduct or practice which does or might constitute a danger to the health, welfare or safety of the patient or the public, or any conduct, practice or condition which does or might impair the ability safely and skillfully to practice medicine.[77]

What such provisions mean in actual practice is another matter. Take malpractice, for example. A physician may be liable in a civil suit for malpractice based on a showing of "ordinary" negligence: failure to exercise the care and skill ordinarily exercised by other physicians. But despite the fact that ordinary negligence may be harmful to the patient, it is doubtful that there is any state in which the act will actually lead to discipline through the licensure mechanism. In those fifteen states that list malpractice among the specific grounds for licensure discipline, the standard is usually phrased "gross malpractice," "gross neglect," "gross carelessness," or "gross incompetence." The practical effect of these provisions, as one study concluded, is that the "disciplinary criteria are . . . analogous to less stringent criminal standards of gross malpractice, which are usually included in state penal statutes."[78] It would appear that Kessel's observation that "once a doctor wins a license to practice, it is almost never revoked unless he is convicted of law-breaking"[79] is scarcely an exaggeration.

Restrictions on Price Competition

The provisions of current licensing laws, then, are consistent with Moore's claim that the purpose of licensing is to restrict entry for the benefit of existing practitioners and are generally inconsistent with the notion that its purpose is to protect the welfare of patients. Medical licensure, however, serves another equally important purpose: It is one of two very powerful weapons that organized medicine can use to control the economic conditions of medical practice. The other weapon — the ability to expel or exclude physicians from county medical societies — will be discussed in detail in chapter 4. These two weapons have been used repeatedly to discipline individual physicians during the long history of the AMA's struggle to manage an effective physicians' cartel.

[77]Ibid., p. 284.

[78]Ibid.

[79]Kessel, "The AMA and the Supply of Physicians," p. 275.

What actions on the part of individual physicians are most threatening to organized medicine? The two principal ones are price cutting and advertising. Economists have long known that controlling entry into a market creates only modest benefits for existing producers. A much more effective and financially lucrative device is the practice of price fixing. But long before the economics of monopoly were fully understood by professional economists, the representatives of organized medicine were ardent advocates of price-fixing schemes. At the first meeting of the AMA in 1847 the representatives not only endorsed fee schedules at the local level but made adherence to such schedules a matter of medical ethics. Chapter II, article 7, section 1, of the *Code of Medical Ethics*, unanimously approved at the 1847 convention, reads as follows:

> Some general rules should be adopted by the faculty, in every town or district, relative to the *pecuniary acknowledgments* from their patients; and it should be deemed a point of honor to adhere to this rule with as much steadiness as varying circumstances will permit.[80]

The existence of such fee schedules, however, does not mean that the AMA endorsed charging every patient the same fee for a specific service. As Professor Kessel has pointed out, the ability to charge high fees to high-income patients and low fees to low-income patients is an essential characteristic of profit-maximizing behavior in the medical marketplace.[81] Kessel furnishes the following quotation by an unnamed, but highly respected surgeon as an example of the position of organized medicine on acceptable pricing policies:

> I don't feel that I am robbing the rich because I charge them more when I know they can well afford it; the sliding scale is just as democratic as the income tax. I operated on two people today for the same condition — one a widow whom I charged $50, the other a banker whom I charged $250. I let the widow set her own fee. I charged the banker an amount which he probably carries around in his wallet to entertain his business friends.[82]

Price discrimination of this sort has often been defended on the grounds that doctors sometimes perform a special type of medical charity: They provide services to poor patients at nominal fees (sometimes at no charge) and finance this charitable activity by collecting

[80] "Code of Medical Ethics."

[81] Kessel, "Price Discrimination in Medicine," p. 22.

[82] The quotation is taken from Max Scham, "Who Pays the Doctor?" *New Republic*, 9 July 1956, p. 10.

higher fees from well-to-do patients. Yet Kessel has shown that economic evidence is inconsistent with the claim of charitable motive. Instead, the evidence supports the notion that physicians engage in price discrimination primarily to maximize income.[83]

Every seller has an economic incentive to price discriminate. Other things being equal, price discrimination always increases profit. Yet in the vast majority of markets for goods and services, price discrimination is not practiced because of the existence of competition. Any attempt to charge a higher price to a special group of customers is thwarted by competitors, who are willing to offer the same good or service at a lower price. Vigorous competition in the medical marketplace might work like this: If the banker patient is being charged a supranormal fee of $250 for an operation by one surgeon, a rival surgeon might compete for the patient by offering a fee of $200. Rather than be a doctor who operates only on widows who set their own fees, the first surgeon might respond by quoting an even lower price. Price competition not only brings down the price paid by the banker, it also tends to raise the price paid by the widow: If doctors are vigorously competing for patients, who will choose to operate on the widow for $50 when a banker can be induced to become a patient at a higher price? Ultimately the widow will discover that in order to find a surgeon willing to operate, she will have to pay as much as bankers are being charged — either that or become a *legitimate object* of genuine charity. Through this process of vigorous price competition uniform prices are established in a market.

The driving force behind the process of price competition is the self-interest of the individual producers. Every producer, including every physician, has an economic incentive to compete for patients on the basis of price. But what is in the self-interest of the physician acting as an individual is definitely not in the interest of physicians as a group. The individual physician must be prevented, or discouraged, from individually pursuing his own self-interest. The pursuit of economic self-interest is the most important obstacle faced by a cartel.

Restrictions on Advertising

To deal with the problem of competition, the AMA, as we have noted, made adherence to a fee schedule an issue of professional ethics. But it also did something else. In order for physicians to compete for patients on the basis of price, there must be some way for the

[83]Kessel, "Price Discrimination in Medicine," p. 23.

physician to communicate to the prospective patient the price he is willing to accept. It is precisely this activity that the AMA sought to eliminate by pronouncing advertising unethical and unprofessional.

In 1961 the licensing laws of forty states specifically defined advertising as unprofessional conduct, and thus grounds for license suspension or revocation.[84] Advertising that is "unprofessional," however, is advertising only of a certain type — that which benefits an individual physician. Advertising that benefits the medical community as a whole is a different matter. Kessel explains the distinction:

> The advertisement of medical services is approved by the medical profession if and only if such advertisements redound to the interest of the medical profession as a whole. Advertisements in this class are, for example, announcements of the availability for sale of Blue Cross-type medical plans. These plans allow their subscribers the choice of any licensed practitioner. Organized medicine consequently takes the position that these advertisements are of benefit to the entire profession. On the other hand, advertisements that primarily redound to the interest of a particular group, for example, advertisements by a closed panel medical group, are frowned upon. Advertisements in this class are, by definition, resorted to only by "unethical" doctors. Why this difference in the position of organized medicine with respect to these two classes of advertising? The approved class, insofar as it achieves its objective, tends to increase the aggregate demand for medical care. On the other hand, the disapproved variety will have the effect of reallocating patients from the profession as a whole to those who advertise. Consequently, advertising in this class constitutes competitive behavior and leads to price cutting. It tends to pit one doctor or one group of doctors against the profession as a whole with respect to shares of the medical care market. Active competition for increased shares of the medical care market by doctors would tend to eliminate price discrimination based on income differences.[85]

Organized medicine has used the twin threat of license suspension or revocation and expulsion from county medical societies on numerous occasions to punish deviant behavior. In the area of advertising, for example, here are some recent cases:[86]

> In Minnesota a gynecologist was warned against making radio and newspaper announcements of his one-week drive to encourage women to obtain pap smears by offering discount prices.

[84]See Forgotson, Roemer, and Newman, p. 281.

[85]Kessel, "Price Discrimination in Medicine," pp. 43–44.

[86]See "The AMA's Bad Case," *New York Times*, 6 December 1978.

In Santa Clara, California, the county medical society prohibited clinic doctors who specialize in preventive industrial medicine from seeking new corporate clients.

In St. Louis the local medical association forced the director of Washington University's sterilization and pregnancy termination clinic to apologize for mailing a brochure describing the center's facilities, even though the brochure was mailed to local physicians.

By far the most important cases of AMA retribution, however, have occurred in those instances where renegade doctors have attempted to form health maintenance organizations and similar types of medical care plans. According to the AMA's Judicial Council, it is "unfair or unethical" for doctors to enter into such contracts "when the compensation . . . is inadequate based on the usual fee for service and class of people in the same community" or "when there is underbidding by physicians in order to secure a contract."[87] We shall examine some of the more notorious of these cases in chapter 5.

The attitude of the AMA toward advertising and price competition is paralleled by the associations of related health practitioners. The code of ethics of the American Dental Association, for example, states:

> It is unethical for a dentist to give lectures or demonstrations before lay groups on a particular technique (such as hypnosis) that he employs in his office.
>
> It is unethical for specialists to furnish so-called patient education pamphlets to general practitioners for distribution to patients where pamphlets, in effect, stress unduly the superiority of the procedures used by specialists. Publication of such so-called patient education material has the effect of soliciting patients.[88]

As an another illustration, consider the rules and regulations of the Michigan Optometric Association in 1969. Eligibility for membership in the association was based on a point system and initial membership required sixty-five points. The point evaluation plan of the association was, in condensed form, as follows:[89]

Total points possible for

Not advertising (refers to media advertising,

[87]Ibid.

[88]Reprinted in Benham, "Guilds and the Form of Competition in the Health Care Sector," p. 459.

[89]Ibid.

telephone book listings, and window displays)	30
Location in a professional or office building (as opposed to "an establishment whose primary public image is one of reduced prices and discount optical outlet")	25
Limiting office identification sign to approved size and content	15
Educational activities (professional meetings and activities)	14
Physical facilities (rooms and laboratory)	8
Functional facilities (equipment)	8
	100

Note that constraints on information account for seventy out of the 100 possible points.

It is important to realize that virtually all of the restrictive practices that we have been describing have either recently been declared illegal or are almost certainly destined to become illegal. A Supreme Court ruling in 1977 declared that actions taken by bar associations to prevent lawyers from advertising their fees violated the free speech rights of lawyers. And the Federal Trade Commission recently issued a trade rule that holds that bans on the advertising of eyeglasses violate federal antitrust laws. Both rulings are likely to be extended to the activities of other professional groups. In addition, in November 1978 an FTC judge ruled that parts of the AMA's code of ethics violate the antitrust laws.[90] The judge concluded that restrictions on advertising, on the solicitation of business, and on contractual arrangements with health care organizations are really intended to protect the incomes of fee-for-service doctors.

Although these rulings may do much to curtail the restrictive practices of the AMA and other professional organizations, the economic effects of the restrictive practices continue to pervade the health care marketplace.

The Economic Effects of Medical Licensure

What are the major economic effects of medical licensure laws? To answer this question completely we would have to imagine what the medical marketplace would be like today if it had evolved over the

[90]The ruling was subsequently upheld on appeal.

last 100 years as a free market rather than as a market subject to tight governmental regulations and controls, a difficult, if not impossible task. Who can begin to guess what a market would be like in which 300,000 practicing physicians and many more potential physicians were free to use their intelligence, their creativity, and their innovative capacities in a truly unfettered, competitive environment? Economic theory, comparisons with other markets, and some limited empirical testing combine to give us a great many insights into how things might be different.

Two of the most important areas in which economic analysis can offer some fairly definitive judgments are physicians' incomes and medical costs. There is a substantial body of evidence showing that the restrictive practices of the AMA have been partially successful in achieving their principle objective: Physicians' incomes are higher then they otherwise would be. Evidence also confirms the existence of a much more substantial effect: Overall medical costs are higher than they otherwise would be. These two effects are produced not only by licensing but also by a number of other regulations and controls.

Other aspects of health care have been affected by medical licensing laws:

Costs of Medical Education One of the unfortunate consequences of the Flexner Report is that medical education has been made artificially expensive. Flexner, as we noted, focused on the inputs of training programs, not on the outputs. Had he merely specified what knowledge and capabilities a physician should have, medical schools would have been left free to experiment and innovate in the search for efficient techniques for achieving these objectives. Instead, he rigidly specified how the training program should be organized. Kessel argues that, as a result, "there was a hiatus of over forty years in the search for better curricula and training methods, and in the utilization of the talents of scientists outside of medical schools for the training of physicians."[91]

In their first year, medical students took anatomy, biochemistry, and physiology. In the second year, they studied microbiology, pathology, and pharmacology. The next two years were spent working in a clinical specialty at a teaching hospital. Often this training pattern was written into state laws.[92] Although there has been some relaxation in these procedures in recent years, Kessel argues that "to

[91]Kessel, "The AMA and the Supply of Physicians," p. 270.

[92]See *The Crisis in Medical Education* (Report on an Exploratory Conference sponsored by the Commonwealth Fund and the Carnegie Corporation of New York), 1966.

this day, there is less variation in medical training than in almost any other field."[93]

One of the principal reasons why there has been so little innovation in medical education is lack of incentive. Those schools that might otherwise have the greatest incentive — new schools and less famous schools — faced the greatest risks. Deviation from the officially sanctioned curriculum was especially risky for these schools because they were vulnerable to decertification. The more renowned schools had less to fear from the licensing authorities but little to gain from innovation. After all, in order to compare the effectiveness of medical training programs it is necessary to compare the effectiveness of their graduates. As Benham notes, such comparisons violate the "guild or professional notion that a uniform high standard of service is always provided."[94]

Furthermore, innovations that reduced the cost and length of the training programs offered by medical schools would almost certainly be resisted by organized medicine. Kessel has asked why "basic science" courses, for example, should be taught in medical schools at all. Such courses are often taught by undistinguished faculties and are often inferior to similar courses that the students have already completed at undergraduate institutions.[95] An obvious answer to Kessel's question is that instruction in theoretical subjects, which are only marginally related to the practice of medicine, lengthens the training program and raises the cost of entry into the profession.

It is no accident that the example provided by organized medicine has been adapted to countless other professions. Many states, for example, make as a prerequisite for a barbering license not less than 1,000 hours of instruction in "theoretical subjects," before actual apprenticeship is begun.[96] When optometry was first licensed in 1901, it was possible to complete the training program in two weeks. The length of training has since increased at a rate of one year per decade. The current training period of eight years represents a 15,600 percent increase over the 79-year period.[97]

[93]Kessel, "The AMA and the Supply of Physicians," p. 269.

[94]Benham, "Guilds and the Form of Competition in the Health Care Sector," p. 453.

[95]Kessel, "The AMA and the Supply of Physicians," p. 277.

[96]See Walter Gelhorn, *Individual Freedom and Governmental Restraints* (Baton Rouge: Louisiana State University Press, 1956), p. 146.

[97]Lee Benham, "Aspects of Occupational Licensure," 42 (St. Louis: Center for the Study of American Business, 1979), p. 14.

The Supply of Minority Physicians One of the least well-known consequences of the Flexner Report was the devastating effect it had on prospective physicians from "minority" groups: blacks, Jews, and women. In 1910 there were seven medical schools that specialized in training black physicians, and between 1900 and 1920 the percentage of black physicians among all physicians increased sharply — from 1.3 percent to 2.0 percent.[98] This trend was expected to have continued as blacks overcame their educational disadvantages, but between 1910 and 1944 the number of black medical schools fell from seven to two, and the percentage of black physicians among all physicians leveled off at its 1910 peak.[99]

Thomas Sowell has shown that a similar phenomenon occurred in many other trades and crafts around the turn of the century.[100] When free markets were allowed to work, it appears that blacks had comparatively little difficulty competing with whites for jobs and positions. Yet the growth of government regulations, the strength of unions, and the demise of proprietary professional schools led to a rationing problem. The demand for certain jobs, such as those in the railroad industry, and the demand for entry into professional schools soon exceeded the supply of positions available. In a free market the decision as to who would get these positions would have been settled by a falling wage or a rising price. In the absence of a free market, these decisions were made by groups and committees.

Since the decision makers on medical school admissions boards could not, or would not, discriminate on the basis of price, they discriminated on other grounds. As Benham explains, "It should not surprise us that the successful members of the subsequent queue looked remarkably similar to those making the admissions decisions."[101] No doubt many of these decision makers reflected the views of Flexner himself. Flexner wrote that "a well-taught negro sanitarian will be immensely useful; an essentially untrained negro wearing an M.D. degree is dangerous" and "the practice of the negro doctor will be limited to his own race."[102]

Similar obstacles were also faced by women and Jews. The number

[98]Kessel, "The AMA and the Supply of Physicians," p. 270.

[99]Ibid.

[100]Thomas Sowell, *Race and Economics* (New York: David McKay Co., 1975).

[101]Benham, "Guilds and the Form of Competition in the Health Care Sector," pp. 455–56.

[102]Flexner, p. 180.

of women in medical schools did not return to pre-Flexner levels until after 1940.[103] And the discrimination against Jewish applicants to medical schools became so intense that one source reports that in the 1930s, 90 percent of Americans studying medicine abroad were Jewish.[104] Not only was discrimination against minority applicants rampant, but when cutbacks in admissions were made in the 1930s minority applicants bore a disproportionate share of the reduction in admissions: The overall reduction in admissions was about 17 percent, but black and Jewish admissions were cut back by about 30 percent.[105]

Efforts to Circumvent Entry Barriers Virtually every economic study on the profitability of medical practice has concluded that admission to a medical school is a valuable economic commodity.[106] There is some disagreement on the size of the economic value of admission, but, with one exception, all students of the subject agree that its value is not zero.[107] In effect, admitting a student to medical school is tantamount to increasing his personal wealth.

It should come as no surprise, then, to learn that prospective students and their families are willing to expend a great deal of effort to secure admission to a medical school. A recent survey of medical admissions procedures concluded that "payments totaling millions of dollars are being made to these schools by parents and friends of prospective students to assure their acceptance." So widespread is the practice that an official at the Department of Health, Education and Welfare recently made the blanket statement that "nearly all the private schools discreetly barter contributions for places in the more sought after graduate schools."[108]

[103]Richard H. Shryock, "Women in American Medicine," *Journal of the American Medical Women's Association* 5 (1950): 377.

[104]Jacob A. Goldberg, "Jews in the Medical Profession — A National Survey," *Jewish Social Studies* 1: 332. For an analysis of some of the reasons for discrimination against Jewish applicants, see Kessel, "Price Discrimination in Medicine," pp. 46–51.

[105]Kessel, "The AMA and the Supply of Physicians," p. 271, n. 18.

[106]For a survey of some of the more important studies in this area, see Frank Sloan and Roger Feldman, "Competition Among Physicians," in *Competition in the Health Care Sector: Past, Present and Future* (Germantown, Md.: Aspen Systems Corporation, 1978), pp. 45–102.

[107]The exception is Cotton Lindsay, "Real Returns to Medical Education," *Journal of Human Resources* (Summer 1973): 331–48. See also Lindsay, "More Real Returns to Medical Education," *Journal of Human Resources* (Winter 1976): 127–30.

[108]Richard Lyons, "Gifts From Parents to 'Buy' Places in Professional Schools on the Rise," *New York Times*, 23 April 1978.

The payments from parents can be quite large. The highest offer reported to date was a covert bid of $250,000 to secure one place in the freshman class at a California medical school. In addition to outright bribery, parents of prospective students have resorted to political pressure and other forms of unethical influence. In one case, a contribution to a medical school in Philadelphia was made on behalf of a student by the Speaker of the lower house of the Pennsylvania legislature, which votes tax funds to support the institution. In another case a student was admitted to the University of California School of Medicine at Davis despite the fact that her admissions score was more than thirty points below the level normally required for acceptance. At the time of her admission, her father-in-law was the chancellor of the university.[109]

One result of the restriction of opportunities for medical education, then, is an admissions system that can at best be described as scandalous. A second is an increase in the number of American students studying medicine abroad. Kessel reports that in the late 1960s the ratio of the number of American enrollments in foreign institutions to the number of foreign enrollments in American institutions ranged from one-fourth to one-thirtieth in business administration, agriculture education, engineering, physical and natural sciences, and economics. In medicine, the ratio of Americans studying abroad to foreigners studying in the United States exceeded three to one for the year 1966.[110]

During the 1970s this trend continued. In recent years estimates reveal between ten and twelve thousand American students studying medicine abroad as compared with sixty-thousand students enrolled in medical schools in the United States.[111] Many of the foreign medical schools apparently provide excellent training, while others appear to be similar to the schools Flexner described seventy years ago.

Proprietary medical schools in the Caribbean, for example, now constitute a booming business, with approximately five thousand U.S. students enrolled. Annual tuition at these schools is often lower than the $6,100 average for U.S. medical schools in 1978 — but so is the standard of training. At one school in the Dominican Republic there is one microscope for every ten students, and each student must purchase his own skeleton for classroom study — usually from the city cemetery for indigents.[112]

109Ibid.

110Kessel, "The AMA and the Supply of Physicians," p. 272.

111Gail Bronson, "New Medical Schools in Caribbean Provoke Controversy in U.S.," *Wall Street Journal*, 19 June 1979.

112Ibid.

TABLE 2.3
Licentiates Representing Additions to the Medical Profession, 1950–1975

Year	Total Newly Licensed	Newly Licensed Graduates of Foreign Medical Schools	Percentage of Foreign Graduates
1950	6,002	308	5.1
1951	6,273	350	5.6
1952	6,885	569	8.3
1953	7,276	685	9.4
1954	7,917	772	9.8
1955	7,737	907	11.7
1956	7,463	852	11.4
1957	7,455	1,014	13.6
1958	7,809	1,166	14.9
1959	8,269	1,626	19.7
1960	8,030	1,419	17.7
1961	8,023	1,580	19.7
1962	8,005	1,357	17.0
1963	8,283	1,451	17.5
1964	7,911	1,306	16.5
1965	9,147	1,528	16.7
1966	8,851	1,634	18.5
1967	9,424	2,081	22.1
1968	9,766	2,185	22.4
1969	9,978	2,307	23.1
1970	11,032	3,016	27.3
1971	12,257	4,314	35.2
1972	14,476	6,661	46.0
1973	16,689	7,419	44.5
1974	16,706	6,613	39.6
1975	16,859	5,965	35.4

SOURCE: Henry R. Mason, *74th Annual Report of Medical Licensure Statistics, Part 2* (Chicago: American Medical Association, 1976), pp. 360–61, tables 6 and 7. Reprinted with the permission of the American Medical Association.

Whatever the defects of medical study abroad, however, foreign medical graduates appear to be able to obtain licenses to practice when they return to the United States. Table 2.3 shows how important these additions to our medical manpower pool have been during the last thirty years. The high-water mark was reached in 1972 when 46 percent of all physicians licensed for the first time were graduates of foreign medical schools.

The Quality of Service Because a major goal of licensing legislation has been to raise the standard of training received by medical students, a natural inference is that medical licensure has led to an improvement in the quality of medical care. There has never been any empirical study to verify this inference,[113] however, and a number of economists, including Milton Friedman,[114] and Frank Sloan and Roger Feldman,[115] have argued that medical licensure actually reduces the quality of care administered to patients.

How could the Flexner reforms have failed to improve the quality of medical practice? First, many of the educational requirements of medical schools have never been shown to relate directly to the quality of the actual practice of medicine. In addition, many of the reforms that did contribute to higher standards of medical care would probably have occurred in any event. As the experience of law schools indicates, improvements in the quality of training do not require Flexner-style legislation.[116] Moreover, as table 2.3 shows, a great many physicians practicing medicine today were not educated in American medical schools. A recent study of state licensing of foreign medical school graduates concluded that variables unrelated to competence or to the adequacy of training (such as citizenship status) are the major determinants of the licensing of these students by state medical boards.[117]

High quality medical care is unlikely to be provided unless doctors have an *incentive.* In general, such an incentive is more likely to prevail where there is intense competition for patients and less likely to prevail where competition is absent.[118] AMA policies that discourage competition in general and advertising in particular discourage improvements in the quality of care that patients receive.

Not only does the AMA discourage comparison of physicians on the basis of the quality of their services, but organized medicine expends a

113Kessel, "The AMA and the Supply of Physicians," p. 273.

114Milton Friedman, *Capitalism and Freedom* (Chicago: University of Chicago Press, 1962), pp. 155–60.

115Sloan and Feldman, p. 46.

116Kessel, "The AMA and the Supply of Physicians," p. 275–76.

117Arlene Goldblatt, Louis Goodman, Stephen Mick, and Rosemary Stevens, "Licensure, Competence and Manpower Distribution," Working Paper W4-37, Yale University Institute for Social Policy Analysis.

118There is some statistical evidence to show that increased competition (as measured by a higher physician-to-population ratio) leads to an increase in such "quality-amenities" as more time spent with patients, shorter waiting times in physicians' offices, greater physician accessibility, etc. See Sloan and Feldman, pp. 79–83.

great deal of effort to see that such information is not collected, and, if collected, not made public. The difficulty of obtaining witnesses to testify for the plaintiff in malpractice cases is so widespread that some lawyers assert that a conspiracy of silence exists. In one case, a patient was unable to hire an expert witness to demonstrate negligence even though the surgeon had left a sponge in his body.[119] Those doctors who do testify can expect retribution. Doctors have been expelled from their county medical societies not only for testifying in malpractice suits[120] but also for merely expressing opinions about the professional competence of their colleagues to their patients.[121]

Physicians are not alone in adhering to the "no criticism" rule. The American Dental Association (ADA), for example, is remarkably explicit about what constitutes "unjust criticism." The code of ethics of the ADA states that

> the dentist has the obligation of not referring disparagingly, orally or in writing, to the services of another dentist to a member of the public. A lack of knowledge of conditions under which the services were offered may lead to unjust criticism and to a lessening of the public's confidence in the dental profession. If there is indisputable evidence of faulty treatment, the welfare of the patient demands that corrective treatment be instituted at once and in such a way as to avoid reflection on the previous dentist or on the dental profession.[122]

What all of this means to the patient was vividly illustrated in a recent study by Nancy Ordway, who went to considerable effort to find some of the most incompetent physicians in the United States and discovered some notorious cases. She then attempted to find out what she could about some of these physicians from the Illinois State Licensing Board, the Illinois State Medical Society, and the American Medical Association. The first two organizations would release no information, and the AMA would release information only on tax evasion and fraud. The AMA refused to release any derogatory informa-

[119]See Kessel, "Price Discrimination in Medicine," p. 45, n. 79.

[120]Melvin Belli, *Ready for the Plaintiff* (New York: Henry Holt, 1956), p. 115. See also Belli, "An Ancient Therapy Still Applied: The Silent Medical Treatment," *Villanova Law Review* 1 (1956).

[121]See "Doctor Fights Expulsion on Slander Charge," *Medical Economics* 32 (December 1954): 269.

[122]American Dental Association, "Principles of Ethics with Advisory Opinions, as revised November 1972," in Jane Clapp, ed., *Professional Ethics and Insignia* (Metuchen, N.J.: Scarecrow Press Inc., 1974), p. 227.

tion about the practice of medicine, even in the cases of physicians who had had their licenses revoked.[123]

Finally, medical licensure has had a deleterious effect on the quality of medical care by sharply reducing heterogeneity in the practice of medicine. The Flexner reforms, according to Kessel, "made medical schools as alike as peas in a pod."[124] The same can be said of the clinical approach of the students who were trained in them. Although the last decade has seen some relaxation in this rigid homogeneity of clinical approach, there is far less variety in the practice of medicine than the state of medical knowledge would seem to warrant. Medical schools, for example, put heavy emphasis on the efficacy of surgical and pharmaceutical intervention. As a consequence, practicing physicians' knowledge of the healing power of nutrition is notoriously limited.[125]

Even in those areas where promising innovations have arisen, medical licensure laws have restricted, or threatened to restrict, their application. The Texas State Board of Medical Examiners, for example, recognizes acupuncture as a legitimate practice of medicine, but requires anyone who administers acupuncture to hold a state medical license. When two Dallas physicians allowed unlicensed oriental attendants to practice acupuncture in their office in 1975, they were placed on ten-year professional probation.[126] The state medical board in Kansas attempted, unsuccessfully, to keep chiropractors from practicing acupuncture.[127] Biofeedback therapy is an innovation that may prove to be highly successful in treating migraine headaches and other illnesses, but at this time an effort is underway to bring this technique under the control of organized medicine, which has little interest in its application.

The Growth in the Number of Other Health Personnel One of the most commonly observed responses to artificial entry barriers in a particular market is the increased production of close substitutes for the good or service being protected. In medicine this response consists of increasingly large numbers of nonphysician health personnel. In

123See Benham, "Guilds and the Form of Competition in the Health Care Sector," p. 462.

124Kessel, "The AMA and the Supply of Physicians," p. 269.

125Benham, "Guilds and the Form of Competition in the Health Care Sector," p. 457.

126"Dallas Physicians' Probation Upheld," *Dallas Times Herald*, 14 February 1979.

127"Kansas Chiropractors Win Legal Battle to Use Acupuncture," *Dallas Times Herald*, 2 December 1979.

1900, for example, the ratio of health personnel trained in other fields to physicians was 0.6. By 1960 that ratio had climbed to 3.7, and it is estimated that in 1980 there will be 4.5 nonphysician professionals for every physician in the United States.[128]

The growth of this ratio is considerably larger if allied health workers with training below the baccalaureate level are counted. In 1900 there was one health worker for each physician. By 1964 the ratio was thirteen health workers for each physician, and by 1975 there were between twenty and twenty-five supportive personnel for each physician. [129] The nature of this development is the subject of chapter 3.

128Roemer, p. 48.

129Ibid., p. 49.

III. CONTROLS ON WHO MAY PRACTICE: NURSES AND OTHER PARAMEDICAL PERSONNEL

All professions are conspiracies against the laity.
George Bernard Shaw, 1906

A startling contrast exists between the market for the services of physicians and the market for the services of professional nurses. In 1979 there were 20 percent fewer medical schools training physicians in the United States than there were in 1900.[1] As table 3.1 shows, however, between 1900 and 1970 the number of nursing schools increased by over 300 percent. The ratio of nurses to doctors, depicted in table 3.2, reflects this difference in educational opportunity. In 1900 there was one professional nurse for every three physicians; by 1970 there were two professional nurses for every physician.

Many other kinds of health personnel besides professional nurses assist physicians these days under such headings as "nurse practitioner," "nurse-midwife," "nurse associate," "nurse clinician," "physician's assistant," "physician's associate," "child-health associate," etc. The economic importance of this cadre of health personnel was accurately summarized in a 1971 message to Congress by President Richard Nixon:

> One of the most promising ways to expand the supply of medical care and to reduce its cost is through a greater use of allied health personnel, especially those who work as physicians' and dentists' assistants, nurse pediatric practitioners, and nurse midwives. Such persons are trained to perform tasks which must otherwise be performed by doctors themselves, even though they do not require the skills of a doctor. Such assistance frees a physician to focus his skills where they are most needed and often allows him to treat many additional patients.[2]

[1]In 1979 there were 125 accredited medical schools in the United States. See Gail Bronson, "New Medical Schools in the Caribbean Provoke Controversy in the U.S.," *Wall Street Journal*, 19 June 1979.

[2]President Richard M. Nixon, "Message to Congress Relative to Building a National Health Strategy," *Congressional Record* 117 (1971): 3319–22.

TABLE 3.1
Professional Nursing Schools: 1880 to 1970[1]

Year	Professional Nursing Schools[2]			Ratio of Nursing Schools to Medical Schools
	Number	Students	Graduates	
1880	15	323	157	0.15
1890	35	1,552	471	0.26
1900	432	11,164	3,456	2.70
1910	1,129	32,636	8,140	8.62
1920	1,755	54,953	14,980	20.65
1930	—	—	—	—
1940	1,311	85,156	23,600	17.03
1950	1,203	98,712	25,790	15.23
1960	1,119	115,057	30,113	12.30
1970	1,328	150,795	43,639	12.41

SOURCE: U.S. Bureau of the Census, *Historical Statistics of the United States, Colonial Times to 1970, Bicentennial Edition, Part 2* (Washington, D.C., 1975), Series B 275–290, pp. 75–76.

[1]Figures for schools and students are for academic session ending in the specified year.

[2]Includes Hawaii and Puerto Rico beginning in 1950 for number and students and beginning in 1952 for graduates.

TABLE 3.2
Active Professional Graduate Nurses: 1910 to 1970

Year	Number	Rate per 100,000 Population	Ratio of Nurses to Physicians[1]
1910	50,500	55	0.37
1920	103,900	98	0.72[2]
1930	214,300	174	1.39[2]
1940	284,200	216	1.62
1950	375,000	249	1.84
1960	504,000	282	1.83
1970	700,000	345	2.01

SOURCE: U.S. Bureau of the Census, *Historical Statistics of the United States, Colonial Times to 1970, Bicentennial Edition, Part 2* (Washington, D.C., 1975), Series B 275–290, pp. 75–76.

[1]Beginning in 1960, physicians include osteopaths.

[2]Census figures are used for number of physicians and may include physicians not in active medical practice.

Historical Background

When President Nixon made that statement in February 1971, the laws of most states severely restricted the right of physicians to delegate the authority to perform "medical acts" to nonphysicians. Typically, medical practice statutes hold that "a person who in any way performs, offers to perform, or holds himself out to the public as performing specific functions — e.g., diagnosing, treating, operating or prescribing for a disease, ailment, pain, or condition — must be licensed as a physician."[3]

Most states have provided exemptions, for example, for persons rendering emergency services, and for medical students, residents, and interns. But aside from these few special categories, the prohibition on the practice of medicine was all-encompassing until fairly recently. In general no "medical act" could be delegated unless specifically provided for by statute. For example, a number of states had specific statutes allowing podiatrists and optometrists to perform independently certain medical acts relating to specific parts of the body, physical therapists to carry out treatments upon referral by physicians, and nurses to administer medications prescribed by a doctor. But these exemptions applied to narrowly defined health personnel and narrowly defined acts. It was possible, for example, for a professional nurse to have legal authority to give innoculations and for an equally qualified practical nurse not to have any such authority.[4]

The language of most medical practice statutes is typically vague and imprecise about what constitutes a "medical act." But in cases testing the legality of the delegation of medical acts, the courts have traditionally given broad readings to the term "practice of medicine." To see just how far the restrictions have gone, consider the case of *Magit* v. *Board of Medical Examiners.*[5] In this case, a California physician had his license revoked for "unprofessional conduct" because he hired unlicensed, foreign-trained anesthesiologists for independent administration of anesthetics. What makes this case especially interesting is that the foreign-trained specialists had previously administered anesthetics under an exemption to the California medical practice act — as employees of a state hospital. In addition, nurses

3Edward Forgotson, Ruth Roemer, and Roger Newman, "Licensure of Physicians," *Washington University Law Quarterly* 332 (1967): 250–51.

4Philip C. Kissam, "Physician's Assistant and Nurse Practitioner Laws: A Study of Health Law Reform," *Kansas Law Review* 24 (1975): 4–5.

557 Cal. 2d. 74, 366 P.2d 816, 17 Cal. Rptr. 488 (1961).

and interns, presumably with less training, regularly administered anesthetics in California under other exceptions to the medical practice act.[6]

The implications of these and other rulings for the practice of medicine have been summarized by Kissam:

> Traditional medical delegation has not included all or even most relatively simple, routine medical acts.... Physical examinations, medical histories, diagnosis and treatment of common illnesses, minor surgery, and decisions to continue or modify prescribed treatment for convalescing or chronically ill patients generally have not been delegated. Furthermore, delegated medical acts have been entrusted only to limited groups of licensed personnel, notwithstanding other nonphysicians' ability to perform the same acts.[7]

Kissam's description is based largely on inferences from statutory law and therefore tells us nothing about how frequently such laws are obeyed. A number of observers believe that violations are widespread. Rayack, for example, asserts that nearly all hospitals have allowed "registered nurses to perform services once performed by doctors, *despite the fact that this is a practice barred by a number of state laws.*"[8]

Both physicians and hospitals, however, face strong disincentives to violate medical practice laws. There is the potential risk of disciplinary proceedings, and, in addition, a number of courts have ruled that violation of a statute raises a presumption of negligence in personal injury suits.[9] A physician who allows an assistant to carry out a procedure that might be considered the "practice of medicine" substantially increases his malpractice jeopardy. In any event, few doubt that violations of statutory law are trivial compared to the enormous potential for the efficient use of paramedical personnel.

During the early 1970s a majority of states began to liberalize their restrictions on the delegation of medical acts. By 1975 at least forty-one states had enacted sixty-six statutes allowing physicians to delegate medical acts innovatively to broadly defined categories of

[6]The court upheld the illegality of the act but ruled that revocation of the physician's license was an abuse of the medical board's discretion.

[7]Kissam, pp. 4–5.

[8]Elton Rayack, *Professional Power and American Medicine: The Economics of the American Medical Association* (Cleveland: World Publishing Co., 1967), p. 127.

[9]Arthur Leff, "Medical Devices and Paramedical Personnel: A Preliminary Context for Emerging Problems," *Washington University Law Review Quarterly* 332 (1967): 387–90.

nonphysicians. Thirty-eight of these statutes authorized delegation to physicians' assistants; twenty-four statutes authorized delegation only to qualified professional nurses, and the remaining four statutes included qualified practical nurses as well.[10] Before looking at the specifics of these recent legal changes, we will look first at their potential economic impact.

The Economic Effects of Legal Restrictions on Paramedical Personnel

Numerous studies have shown that trained nurses and physicians' assistants can competently perform a great many medical procedures. The nonphysicians studied have ranged from high-school graduates with four to six weeks of training to professional nurses. The delegation of tasks studied has ranged from the diagnosis of certain well-defined medical complaints to independent general practice, with complex problems referred to appropriate physicians.

For example, a decision must be made as to whether an ailment of the upper respiratory tract is a symptom of a common cold, a common throat infection, or a more serious disorder. One study showed that both nurses and other trained nonphysicians were capable of making this decision as competently as physicians.[11] Recent studies also show that nonphysicians can perform as competently as physicians in a wide variety of other procedures, including diagnostic and treatment judgments and treatment modifications for common illnesses.[12]

Two other studies illustrate just how far the delegation of medical tasks might be carried. In the first, pediatric nurses are able to give

10Kissam, p. 1.

11Greenfield, Bragg, McGraith, and Blackburn, "Upper-Respiratory Tract Complaint/Protocol for Physician-Extenders," *Archives of Internal Medicine* 133 (1974): 294–99.

12See Bessman, "Comparisons of Medical Care in Nurse Clinician and Physician Clinics in Medical School Affiliated Hospitals," *Journal of Chronic Disorders* 27 (1974); Charles, Stimson, Mausier, and Good, "Physician's Assistants and Clinical Algorithms in Health Care Delivery," *Annals of Internal Medicine* 81 (1974); Charney and Kitzman, "The Child-Health Nurse (Pediatric Nurse Practitioner) in Private Practice," *New England Journal of Medicine* 285 (1971); Komaroff, Black, Flately, Knopp, Reiffen, and Sherman, "Protocol for Physician Assistants — Management of Diabetes and Hypertension," *New England Journal of Medicine* 290 (1974); Lewis, Resnik, Schmidt, and Waxman, "Activities, Events and Outcomes in Ambulatory Patient Care," *New England Journal of Medicine* 280 (1969); Runyon, "The Memphis Chronic Disease Program: Comparisons in Outcome and the Nurse's Extended Role," *Journal of the American Medical Association* 231 (1975).

"total care" to more than 75 percent of all children who come to pediatric clinics. In another, professional nurses with three months of additional training are allowed to maintain an independent, family practice. The nurses are able to handle competently about two-thirds of all cases, referring the remaining third to other physicians.[13]

Delegation of diagnostic authority, of course, always carries with it some risk. Even if a nurse can give innoculations as competently as a physician, she is unlikely to be able to deal as well as the physician with clinically common emergencies, such as anaphylactic shock. These risks, however, do not seem out of line with many other risks that are routinely taken both by patients and their doctors. Patients, for example, often take risks by choosing to leave their conditions undiagnosed. Physicians and hospitals take a great many risks under the present exemptions to medical practice acts. For example, interns, who are often not licensed during their internships, are sometimes given critical responsibilities, including spot diagnosis, prescription and treatment, minor surgery, obstetrical deliveries, lumbar punctures, etc. Nurses are often permitted to administer anesthesia, and critical hematological and general pathological procedures are frequently carried out by nonphysician technologists or technicians.[14]

In addition, it may well be that many patients will come to prefer treatment by trained nonphysicians to treatment by physicians. It is a common joke among patients that shots given by nurses hurt less than shots given by doctors. Recent evidence gives some support to this folk wisdom by showing that physicians' assistants and nurses provide more personal attention to patients than physicians do in comparable situations.[15]

The enormous potential inherent in the unutilized and underutilized services of nurses and other nonphysician personnel was the major reason why the Duke University Medical Center began its Physician's Assistants Program in 1965. During the Vietnam War, about 30,000 medics were being discharged annually from the armed services.[16] Many of them had had extensive health care services experience, and

[13]Spitzer, Sackett, Sibley, Roberts, Tech, Gent, Kergin, Hackett, and Olynich, "The Burlington Randomized Trial of the Nurse Practitioner," *New England Journal of Medicine* 290 (1974): 251–56.

[14]Leff, pp. 380–81.

[15]See Bessman, Lewis et al., and Runyon et al.

[16]Rick J. Carlson, "Health Manpower Licensing and Emerging Institutional Responsibility for the Quality of Care," *Law and Contemporary Problems* 35 (1970): 853.

the Duke program was specifically designed to include this group. The Pediatric Nurse Program at the University of Colorado was also established in 1965 to meet another need. At any one time a large number of trained nurses are not practicing,[17] perhaps in part because of the lack of professional challenge, underutilization, and low pay. Both of these programs were designed to train nonphysicians to handle enhanced delegated authority in the delivery of medical services. Since 1965 numerous other programs have been established with similar objectives.

The economic importance of these programs and the related relaxation of licensing restrictions on paramedical personnel can be quickly appreciated by considering a few economic statistics. For example, compare the cost of training a nurse to handle competently additional medical acts with the cost of training a physician to handle those same tasks. One study found that the total cost of training a professional nurse as a pediatric nurse practitioner (capable of additional delegated authority) was only $1,755 in 1972 — far less than the cost of training a physician that year.[18] Consider also the difference in fees: On the average, physicians' incomes today are from four to six times as high as the incomes of professional nurses.[19]

Of course, if nurses receive extra training they will be more productive, and their market value will rise. In addition, evidence suggests that effective utilization of nurse practitioners will allow employer-physicians to increase their incomes as well. One recent study found that the use of physicians' assistants trained in the Duke University program raised the productivity (measured by the number of cases handled per week) of physicians by 40 to 70 percent.[20] Another study found that use of physicians' assistants may raise physician produc-

17A. Sadler, B. Sadler, and A. Bliss, *The Physician's Assistant - Today and Tomorrow* (New Haven: Yale University Press, 1972), fig. 2, p. 60.

18Yankover, Tripp, Andrews, and Connelly, "The Cost of Training and the Income Generation Potential of Pediatric Nurse Practitioners," *Pediatrics* 49 (1972): 878, 881. The Association of American Medical Colleges estimated that medical school costs in 1979 averaged about $17,000 per year per student. See Rick Jaroslovsky, "Too Many Doctors? Medical Schools May Face Cutback," *Wall Street Journal*, 15 March 1979.

19Kissam, p. 6. The AMA's estimates for average net incomes of physicians by specialty ranged from a little over $40,000 for pediatricians and general practitioners to more than $58,000 for surgeons in 1973. That same year, the average annual salaries of general duty registered nurses in public hospitals in twenty-one major cities ranged from $8,500 to $11,000.

20I. R. Pondy, "Physician Assistants' Productivity: An Interim Report," (Duke University School of Business Administration, January 1971).

tivity by 49 to 74 percent, depending on the extent of delegation. The study concluded that a physician employing a single qualified physician's assistant can potentially increase his income from fees by 160 percent while increasing total labor costs by only $141 per week.[21] Subsequent work has demonstrated that the cost of physicians' services fall substantially when physicians' assistants are effectively used in group practices.[22]

Expanded delegation of authority to qualified nonphysicians is also a promising solution to the problem of the so-called under-doctored areas. In 1970 more than one-third of the counties in the United States had a physician-population ratio less than one-third the national average. No private physicians were found in 130 of these counties. Similar conditions existed in low-income, inner-city areas.[23] The government's current solution to this problem is to make two years of service in an under-doctored area a requirement for medical students whose medical education was financed by the federal government in return for a two-year commitment to serve in the National Health Service Corps. The government is also offering high fees to young doctors who will volunteer to practice in these areas. In 1978, for example, a volunteer could get $46,000 a year in return for practicing in an under-doctored area.[24]

The government's solution is expensive and probably quite wasteful — most corps physicians are not expected to remain in the areas where they are practicing once their two-year hitch is up, and therefore by the time they become personally familiar with most of their patients, they will be replaced by another physician. Relaxation of licensing restrictions, by contrast, enlarges the potential supply of medical services enormously. It is expected that many trained physicians' assistants will be far more willing to practice permanently in under-doctored areas than physicians currently are and can be induced to do so at a much lower price.

Liberalization of licensing restriction on nonphysician health per-

[21]Kenneth Smith, Marianne Miller, and Fredrick Golladay, "An Analysis of the Optimal Use of Inputs in the Production of Medical Services," *Journal of Human Resources* 7 (1972): 218–23.

[22]Fredrick Golladay, Marilyn Manser, and Kenneth Smith, "Scale Economies in the Delivery of Medical Care: A Mixed Integer Programming Analysis of Efficient Manpower Utilization," *Journal of Human Resources* 9 (1974): 50–62.

[23]Nixon, p. 3122.

[24]Ronald Sullivan, "U.S. to Send 20 to 50 Doctors to Poorer Sections in New York," *New York Times*, 31 January 1978.

sonnel, then, promises a great many economic benefits. Health care can be delivered more efficiently and at a lower cost, with only a modest increase in risk for patients. For literally thousands of nonphysicians, opportunities will be created to earn higher incomes and pursue more satisfying jobs. Individual physicians can look forward to enhanced productivity and, hence, higher incomes. Liberalization of licensing restrictions also promises to be a more effective and less costly way of ameliorating the health care problems of underdoctored areas. By contrast, failure to enact more liberal licensing laws commits us to a course that denies us these benefits.

Why then would anyone oppose licensing changes that permit more delegation of authority to nonphysician personnel? And why did we wait until the decade of the 1970s to make those changes that have been made? The answer is that liberalized licensing legislation potentially threatens the incomes of practicing physicians, taken as a group. Although the ability to delegate authority innovatively promises to raise the productivity, and, thus, the income of the individual physician-employer, these gains can be realized in general only if the physician expands the size of his practice. Kissam has explained the economic consequences for the profession as a whole:

> Expanded medical delegation seems likely to increase the effective supply of physician services and to introduce into physician markets increased opportunities and pressures for effective economic competition.... Physicians and profit-making medical institutions are likely to discover that they can increase their incomes through the employment of trained assistants, but only if their practices are substantially expanded. Similarly, not-for-profit private and public medical institutions may find it more economical to open or expand ambulatory services by employing trained assistants. Such expansions of service may be possible only if patients can be drawn away from other physicians and institutions through increasing price and nonprice competition.[25]

The position of the AMA on liberalizing licensing restrictions has been a bit schizophrenic. Prior to 1970 most of the important court cases on the issue of delegated authority pitted a physician against a state licensing board that usually represented the viewpoint of organized medicine. The AMA favored tight restrictions over the licensing of the physicians themselves. In an apparent reversal of policy, however, the AMA's House of Delegates in December 1970 recommended that state medical practice acts be amended "to remove any

[25]Kissam, p. 17.

barriers to increased delegation of tasks to allied health personnel by physicians."[26]

As more and more states began to follow this recommendation, however, the concern of organized medicine began to grow. In its December 1971 meeting, the AMA's House of Delegates recommended that new legislation be written so that the physician's assistant "will not supplant the doctor in the sphere of decision-making required to establish a diagnosis and plan therapy."[27] The view that only the physician should make diagnoses and plan therapy was apparently motivated by a desire to ensure that nonphysician personnel merely *supplement* rather than *substitute* for physicians' services.

By the time the AMA House of Delegates convened their meeting in June 1972, the representatives of organized medicine were showing much deeper concern. At that meeting the delegates concluded that expanded authority should not be delegated to physicians' assistants who are employees of hospitals or who are employees of full-time, salaried, hospital-based physicians.[28] The delegates went on to recommend that state licensing laws require delegated authority to be approved by state licensing boards on a case by case basis.[29] If accepted, this proposal would mean that before a physician could delegate authority to an assistant, he would be required to submit for the licensing board's approval a job description of the proposed functions of that assistant. The House of Delegates also recommended that reimbursements for the services of physicians' assistants made by private and public insurance plans be limited to those services that had individual licensing board approval, thereby inviting the support of third-party payers for the AMA's recommended form of legislation.[30]

Recent Trends in Licensing Legislation

Recent laws authorizing physicians to delegate medical acts to assistants can be classified as either "nurse practitioner acts" or "physi-

[26]"Licensure of Health Occupations, Recommendation (a)" (prepared by the AMA Council on Health Manpower; adopted by the AMA House of Delegates, December 1970), reprinted in Sadler, Sadler, and Bliss, n. 9, Appendix I.

[27]AMA House of Delegates, *Essentials of an Approved Educational Program for the Assistant to the Primary Care Physician* 1 (December 1971), p. 1.

[28]AMA House of Delegates, *Employment of Physicians' Assistants,* June 1972. A similar position was taken by the American Hospital Association in November 1970.

[29]AMA Board of Trustees, Report 2, *Guidelines for Compensating Physicians for Services of Physicians Assistants* 2, Recommendation 1 (approved by the AMA House of Delegates, June 1972), p. 1.

[30]Ibid., Recommendation 4, p. 2.

cians' assistants acts." The latter refer generally to nonphysician personnel who are not professional or practical nurses. These two types of statutes can also be classified as "simple authorization statutes" or "regulatory statutes." In general, regulatory statutes establish some form of administrative control over the delegation of authority and frequently place this control in the hands of state licensing boards. Simple authorization statues, on the other hand, do not allow for administrative regulation.[31]

The most recent general survey of these statutes was conducted by Kissam in 1975.[32] The legal environment was generally in a state of flux in the five years prior to Kissam's study, and therefore it seems reasonable to suppose that a great many changes have been enacted in the five years since. Nonetheless, Kissam's survey provides a compelling case for the conclusion that state legislatures these days are being influenced far more by the pressures of special interest groups than by the desire to achieve efficient, low-cost health care delivery. As Kissam explains:

> Much of the new legislation is incomplete and unduly restrictive and . . . consequently the maximum feasible amount of expanded delegation may not be achieved. These failures may be explained by two basic factors. Legislators and administrators appreciate easily articulated and administered standards regulating the quality of care, but in many cases these standards unduly restrict expanded delegation. *A more significant factor has been the political power of physicians and other health professionals, whose interests are well served by maintenance of strict controls over expanded medical delegation.*[33]

As an example of Kissam's contention, consider the apparent influence of the AMA on recent legislation. If the objectives outlined by the AMA's House of Delegates in June 1972 are to be achieved, regulatory statutes are clearly preferable to simple authorization statutes. Between 1969 and 1972 a number of states passed statutes in simple authorization form. Since 1972, however, only one state has adopted a simple authorization physician's-assistant statute. Meanwhile, one state has repealed its simple authorization statute and two others have replaced theirs with regulatory statutes. In addition, twelve of the seventeen nurse practitioner statutes passed since 1972 have been regulatory statutes.[34] The AMA has also apparently been

31See Kissam, pp. 26–27.

32Ibid.

33Ibid., p. 2. (Emphasis added.)

34Ibid., pp. 32–33.

quite successful in limiting the role of the physician's assistant in hospitals. As of 1975 at least thirteen states prohibited hospitals from employing physicians' assistants, and several other states showed indications that their regulatory bodies were inclined to adopt similar restrictions.[35]

The AMA is by no means the only organized group with an economic interest in the new legislation. An equally important interest is represented by organized nursing, although the economic interests of nurses in liberalizing medical licensing laws are conflicting. On the one hand, nurses have much to gain by legislation that allows expanded delegation to nurses themselves because such delegation, as we have noted, will increase their market value. On the other hand, nurses have correctly feared that their economic interests will be harmed by legislation that allows the duties of physicians' assistants who are not nurses to overlap with the duties of nursing.[36]

Organized nursing has at times either opposed the enactment of physician's-assistant statutes or tried to restrict their provisions. The New York State Nurses' Association, for example, was the major opponent to enactment of a physician's-assistant statute in New York in 1970 and caused its defeat. When the act passed the following year, the nurses were successful in inserting a provision that prohibited physicians' assistants from performing "duties specifically delegated by law to those persons licensed as allied health professionals." In other states organized nursing has promoted statutes that authorized expanded delegation only to registered nurses, with regulatory controls placed in the hands of state nurse-licensing boards. These boards are effectively controlled by state nurses' associations in a manner similar to the way state medical associations control medical licensing boards.[37] The fact that nurses are far better organized than potential physicians' assistants may help explain why there are so many more simple authorization statutes for nurses than there are for physicians' assistants.

Organized nursing is not the only force with which physicians' assistants have had to contend. As of 1973 optometric associations

[35]Ibid., p. 55.

[36]See American Nurses Association Board of Directors, "The American Nurses Association Views the Emerging Physician's Assistant," 17 December 1971; and New York State Nurses Association Board of Directors, "New York State Nurses Association's Statement on the Physician's Associate and Specialist's Assistant," 31 January 1972. Both are reprinted in Sadler, Sadler, and Bliss, Appendices E and F.

[37]Kissam, pp. 19–20.

had been successful in inserting clauses in the statutes of ten states that prohibited physicians' assistants from providing optometric services. Recent technological breakthroughs have made it possible for eye refractions and eyeglass prescriptions to be determined by sophisticated mechanical devices. These new devices apparently threaten the existence of professionally trained optometrists.[38]

Other groups have also sought to restrict the scope of the functions that can be legally delegated to physicians' assistants. As of 1973 statutes prohibited physicians' assistants from practicing dentistry in six states; from practicing dental hygiene in five states; from practicing pharmacology in five states; and from practicing chiropractics in two states.[39]

A natural expectation is that as physicians' assistants become more numerous and better organized, they too will become a potent political force. For example, New York is one of the few states that requires physicians' assistants to have two years of academic training in order to provide primary care. It is hardly a coincidence that the Brooklyn Hospital–Long Island University Physician's Associate Program, one of the major forces responsible for passage of the New York law, offers a two-year training program.[40]

If the precedent set by other professions is followed, we can expect to see a great deal more legislation lengthening the training period for physicians' assistants, despite the fact that evidence indicates that such extensions do little to improve their market value.[41] Indeed, a reasonable extrapolation of the past into the future suggests that

> the new legislation may encourage the development of categories of physicians' assistants and nurse practitioners with specified qualifications and duties. Such groups may be expected to have the traditional economic interest of licensed occupations in controlling supply by obtaining legislative rules that prohibit all persons without minimum like qualifications from performing a specified range of medical acts.[42]

38Winston Dean, "State Legislation for Physician's Assistants: Review and Analysis," *Health Services Reports* 88 (January 1973): 8.

39Ibid.

40Kissam, n. 66, p. 11.

41See Richard Scheffler, "The Market for Paraprofessionals: The Physician Assistant," *Quarterly Review of Economics and Business* 41 (October 1974): 58.

42Ibid., pp. 18–19.

IV. CONTROLS ON THE FORM OF DELIVERY: THE HOSPITAL

Now, what I contend is that my body is my own, at least I have always so regarded it. If I do harm through my experimenting with it, it is I who suffer, not the state.

Mark Twain

It is well known among students of the American health care system that the Flexner Report led to the demise of the proprietary medical school. Some writers have even pointed out that this demise was a explicit goal of the American Medical Association.[1] But to my knowledge, no one has explained why this development was so important to the AMA's objective of establishing an effective physician's cartel.

Nonprofit educational institutions tend to be dominated by the interests and goals of their faculties.[2] In general, the natural inclination of these faculties is to pursue knowledge as an end in itself. Rarely will faculty members compare the cost of additional training with its "commercial" benefit. The implicit assumption is that more and higher quality training is, like knowledge, a desirable end in itself, regardless of its economic benefit. The natural inclination of these faculties, then, dovetails nicely with the traditional AMA interest in lengthening the period of a physician's training and raising the cost of education.

Proprietary medical schools, on the other hand, will inevitably be dominated by the owner's interests in maximizing profit. To the degree that medical schools sell services to their clients (medical students), they have an incentive to provide additional training only to the extent that such training produces an economic benefit to the student that exceeds its cost. Proprietary schools also have an interest in shortening the length of the training period and in minimizing the cost of training. The objectives of proprietary medical schools, therefore, conflict dramatically with the goals of the AMA.

1See, for example, Ronald Hamowy, "The Early Development of Medical Licensing Laws in the United States, 1975–1900," *Journal of Libertarian Studies* 3, no. 1 (1979): 75.

2For an explanation of why these institutions come to be dominated by their faculties, see Henry G. Manne, *The Political Economy of Modern Universities* (Menlo Park, Calif.: The Institute for Humane Studies, 1975).

A similar principle applies to another, often neglected, phenomenon: the demise of the proprietary hospital. Control over the nation's hospitals is an important and powerful weapon in the hands of organized medicine. This control has made it possible for the AMA to supervise the practice of medicine by those physicians who have successfully overcome the barriers to entry into the profession. The professional goals of organized medicine, however, are in natural conflict with the desire of the individual physician to maximize income and with the desire of the individual hospital to maximize profit.

The experience of other attempts to form successful cartels both in markets for goods and in markets for professional services suggests that AMA control over physicians' professional behavior would be difficult, if not impossible, were hospital services provided exclusively by profit-maximizing institutions, vigorously competing in the marketplace. A market dominated by nonprofit, government-owned hospitals, however, is much more amenable to the achievement of the goals of organized medicine. The demise of the proprietary hospital, therefore, is of enormous economic significance.

The Proprietary Hospital

It is not known precisely how many proprietary hospitals existed around the turn of the century, but by one estimate approximately 56 percent of all hospitals were proprietary in 1910, the year the Flexner report was released.[3] As table 4.1 shows, this percentage declined substantially during the post-Flexner period. For-profit hospitals comprised only 36 percent of the total hospital stock in 1938 and fell to a mere 11 percent by 1968.

What accounts for this trend? Is it possible that nonproprietary hospitals have been able to provide better quality services at a lower cost than the proprietary institutions? There is no evidence to support this contention, nor is there evidence to support the view that the decline of the proprietary hospital was the result of genuine market competition. Instead, there is every reason to believe that the dominance of nonprofit institutions in the market for hospital services is an artificial phenomenon, produced by government intervention in the market for hospital services.

A commonly held view is that the profit orientation of the pro-

[3]The method of estimation is described in Bruce Steinwald and Duncan Neuhauser "The Role of the Proprietary Hospital," *Law and Contemporary Problems* (Autumn 1970), pp. 818–19.

TABLE 4.1
Proprietary Hospitals, 1873–1968

Year	Total Number of Hospitals of All Types	Number of Proprietary Hospitals	Proprietary Hospitals as a Percent of Total Hospitals
1873	178		
1878	442		
1903	2500		
1909	4359		
1910	—	2441 (*est.*)	56 (*est.*)
1914	5047		
1918	5323		
1923	6830		
1928	6852	2435	36
1938	6166	1681	27
1941	6358	1584	25
1946	6125	1076	18
1950	6788	1218	18
1956	6966	981	14
1960	6876	856	12
1966	7160	852	12
1968	7137	769	11

SOURCE: Bruce Steinwald and Duncan Neuhauser, "The Role of the Proprietary Hospital," *Law and Contemporary Problems*, Autumn 1970, table 1, p. 819. Reprinted by permission.

prietary hospital may tempt it to cut costs by reducing the quality of services offered.[4] This view is often supported by casual empiricism. In some parts of the country, such as New York City, it is widely believed that doctors who practice in proprietary hospitals do so because they cannot gain admitting privileges at the more renowned voluntary

[4]See, for example, Edward Forgotson, Ruth Roemer, and Roger Newman, "Innovations in the Organization of Health Services: Inhibiting vs. Permissive Regulation," *Washington University Law Quarterly*, 1967, pp. 400–13. For a representative sample of physician's opinion on the difference in quality between proprietary and nonproprietary hospitals, see Milton Roemer, A. Taher Moustafa, and Carl E. Hopkins, "A Proposed Hospital Quality Index: Hospital Death Rates Adjusted for Case Severity," *Health Services Research* 3 (1968): 96–118; Duncan Neuhauser and Fernand Turcotte, "Costs and Quality of Care in Different Types of Hospitals," *The Annals of the American Academy of Political And Social Science* 399 (January 1972): 50–61; Milton C. Maloney, Roy E. Trussel, and Jack Elinson, "Physicians Choose Medical Care: A Sociometric Approach to Quality Appraisal," *Journal of the American Public Health Association* 50, no. 11 (November 1960): 1678; and Herbert Bynder, "Doctors as Patients: A Study of the Medical Care of Physicians and Their Families," *Medical Care* 6, no. 2 (March/April 1968): 157.

hospitals.[5] Presumably they cannot gain admitting privileges because they are less competent than the doctors who do secure those privileges.[6]

To compare a representative proprietary hospital with large, famous teaching hospitals is, however, highly misleading. The typical proprietary hospital is smaller and offers a narrower range of services than the typical voluntary hospital, for reasons to be discussed below. When proprietaries have been compared with nonprofit hospitals of similar size, offering comparable services, no obvious quality differences have been shown to exist. One study, for example, found that when similar size hospitals are compared, there is little difference between the percentage of proprietary and nonproprietary hospitals that are accredited.[7]

There is no evidence to indicate that proprietary hospitals are inferior in quality. In fact, some proprietary hospitals were created in order to improve the quality of care offered to the public. The End Result Hospital, founded by Ernest Codman in 1911, is one example. Codman started his own proprietary hospital after he quit Massachusetts General Hospital in disgust over the lack of quality control.[8]

The issue of cost is a bit more complicated. A number of researchers have been misled by focusing on a single statistic: average cost per patient per day.[9] Looking at this statistic alone gives the impression that proprietary hospitals are less efficient than nonproprietaries. What matters, however, is not the cost per day, but the *total cost* of a stay in the hospital. A patient who pays $100 for a single day in the hospital is better off financially than a patient receiving the same treatment who pays $50 per day and stays for three days.

The average length of stay for a specific condition varies widely among hospitals, and many health economists believe that length of stay is the most important indicator of a hospital's efficiency. In

[5]See Steinwald and Neuhauser, p. 829.

[6]I use the term "voluntary" for nonprofit, private hospitals because it is the convention. In fact, however, proprietary hospitals are also completely voluntary both in inception and in operation.

[7]See Steinwald and Neuhauser, p. 821.

[8]See Ernest A. Codman, *A Study in Hospital Efficiency* (Boston: privately printed, 1916 or 1917), and Ernest A. Codman, *The Shoulder* (New York: G. Miller & Co. Medical Publishers, Inc., 1934), Introduction and Epilogue.

[9]See, for example, Steinwald and Neuhauser, p. 837; and J. Pettengill, "The Financial Position of Private Community Hospitals, 1961–71," *Social Security Bulletin*, November 1973, pp. 3–11.

general, the more the efficient the hospital, the shorter the average length of stay will be. Victor Fuchs explains why:

> An important determinant [of length of stay] is the efficiency with which the staff carries out the necessary diagnostic and therapeutic procedures. Are there delays in conducting tests and taking X-rays? Do these have to be repeated because of errors? Are operating rooms available when needed? Do patients linger longer than necessary simply because their physicians are away or have forgotten to discharge them? Adverse side effects of drugs, tests, and surgery also frequently increase the length of stay. One study of hospitalization for neurosurgery found that post-operative infection, which occurred in 17 percent of the cases, extended the average stay an additional eighteen days.[10]

Of course, length-of-stay statistics are not foolproof indicators of efficiency. One way a hospital can reduce the average length of stay is to discharge patients prematurely, thus endangering their health. In addition, the "optimal" length of stay for a certain treatment may vary radically from patient to patient because of important differences in their medical conditions. Nonetheless, numerous studies have confirmed that, on the average, patients spend too much time in hospitals, not too little, and that the average length of stay for a great many surgical procedures can be substantially reduced with no discernible adverse effects.[11] In fact, one specialist maintains that early discharge after surgery is actually better for a patient's health.[12]

One of the ironies of hospital economics, however, is that a lower average length of stay tends to raise the average daily cost per patient. One of the reasons is that patients who remain in the hospital long after an operation is performed are typically incurring only the "hotel" cost of the hospital — room and board. As the treatment costs are spread out over more and more days of recuperation, average cost per day becomes lower. On the other hand, early hospital discharge causes the treatment costs to be spread over only a few days of hospital stay. A second reason for this phenomenon is that long lengths of stay make it easier for hospital administrators to keep occupancy rates up. With high occupancy rates, the fixed costs of the hospital are spread over more patients per time period. With shorter stays and a more rapid

[10]Victor Fuchs, *Who Shall Live?* (New York: Basic Books, 1974), p. 98.

[11]Ibid.

[12]Paul T. Lahti, "Early Post-Operative Discharge of Patients from the Hospital," *Surgery* 63 (March 1968): 410–15.

TABLE 4.2

A Comparison of Total Hospital Costs for an Average Hospital Stay at Proprietary, Voluntary and Government Hospitals, 1965–67[1]

Type of Hospital[2]	Average Cost per Day[3]	Average Length of Stay (Days)	Total Cost
Proprietary hospitals	$47.29	6.68	$314.56
Voluntary hospitals	43.68	7.79	338.71
Government hospitals	43.60	7.52	327.87

SOURCE: Based on data presented in Ralph Berry, "Cost and Efficiency in the Production of Hospital Services," *Health and Society—Milbank Memorial Fund Quarterly*, Summer 1974, pp. 291–313.

[1]Based on predicted average cost per patient per day and actual average-length-of-stay statistics.

[2]All hospitals are short-term general hospitals. Approximately six thousand hospitals were sampled.

[3]Average cost per day was adjusted for differences among hospitals in size, quality of services, scope of services offered, input costs, and other variables affecting hospital efficiency.

turnover of patients, keeping occupancy rates high is a more difficult task, requiring a more efficient hospital administration.[13]

The importance of these general principles is illustrated in table 4.2. The estimates of average cost per patient per day were based on a study of over 6,000 American hospitals. These estimates have been adjusted for differences among hospitals in approximately thirty to forty different types of services offered, as well as for differences in hospital size, labor costs, construction costs, etc., in order to make them as comparable as possible. The first column of figures in table 4.2 shows that if a proprietary, a voluntary, and a governmental hospital were offering identical services and were identical in every other respect (except for organizational form), the average cost per patient per day would be $3.61 higher in the proprietary hospital than in the voluntary hospital and $3.68 higher than in the governmental hospital.

The second column of figures in table 4.2 shows that proprietary hospitals have been the most successful in reducing the average length of stay. The third column of table 4.2 indicates the total cost of a hospital stay, based on the numbers in the first two columns. As the

[13]Fuchs, pp. 99–100.

data reveal, the total cost of treatment in the proprietary hospital is $24.15 cheaper than in the voluntary hospital and $13.31 cheaper than in the governmental hospital.

Of course, if all three types of hospitals were identical in every respect other than organizational form, it is possible that no differences in average length of stay would exist. However, the conclusion reached by Ralph Berry, the author of the study from which these numbers were taken, is instructive: "It is quite likely that proprietary hospitals utilize their facilities more intensively per patient per day and consequently incur a higher cost per patient day but a lower total cost per patient, other things equal."[14]

This insight should not be surprising, because the owners of proprietary hospitals have excellent incentives to strive for efficiency. To the degree that efficiency is achieved, the owners of the proprietary hospital will reap its full economic rewards. To the degree that inefficiency prevails, the owners will bear the full costs. The managers of voluntary hospitals, although not necessarily indifferent to efficiency, do not have similar incentives. The managers of these institutions will neither reap the full rewards, nor bear the full costs of their decisions if the institutions become more or less efficient.[15]

The puzzling thing about table 4.2 is the numbers for government hospitals. Both economic theory and empirical evidence suggest that government-run organizations tend to be less efficient than private organizations, including nonprofit institutions. Comparisons of Veterans Administration hospitals and voluntary hospitals, for example, show that the average length of stay for a wide variety of procedures is twice as long in the former than in the latter.[16] Comparisons between government-owned hospitals in the British National Health Service and voluntary hospitals in the United States show similar results.[17]

A possible answer to the puzzle has been suggested by Charles Phelps

[14]Ralph Berry, "Cost and Efficiency in the Production of Hospital Services," *Health and Society — Milbank Memorial Fund Quarterly*, Summer 1974, p. 306.

[15]For a discussion of the economic incentives facing the managers of proprietary, nonprofit, and governmental institutions, see Armen Alchian and William Allen, *Exchange and Production: Competition, Coordination and Control*, 2d. ed. (Belmont, Calif.: Wadsworth, 1977), chap. 9.

[16]See Cotton Lindsay, *Veterans Administration Hospitals: An Economic Analysis of Government Enterprise* (Washington, D.C.: American Enterprise Institute for Public Policy Research, 1975), p. 47.

[17]Cotton Lindsay, *Government in Medicine: The British Experience* (Nutley, N.J.: Roche Laboratories, 1979).

in another context. Phelps argues that in the 1960s (when Berry's study was done) state and local government hospitals provided free care to a disproportionate share of charity patients. He concludes that since the government hospitals did not really compete for these patients, they were provided with a lower quality of care. Patients admitted to these hospitals as charity cases were frequently treated as "teaching patients" for physicians in training. In government hospitals surgery was often performed by residents and interns, with medical students assisting, rather than by the attending staff, with interns and residents assisting, as in private teaching hospitals.[18]

Phelps argues that since the advent of Medicare and Medicaid, however, "charity" patients have had considerably more choice about the hospitals they patronize. As a consequence, state and local governmental hospitals have had to increase the quality of their services in order to retain their share of patients. The evidence seems to bear out this theory. In 1965 governmental hospitals had 7 percent *fewer* employees per patient day than voluntary hospitals. By 1977, however, governmental hospitals had 5 percent *more* employees per patient day. These facts imply that costs have been rising much faster in governmental hospitals than in voluntary hospitals.[19]

The Competitive Disadvantages of Proprietary Hospitals

If there is no evidence that proprietary hospitals offer lower quality services or have higher costs than their rivals, then what explains the demise of the proprietary hospital since 1910? The answer is government policy. Traditionally, proprietary hospitals have struggled to compete within a hostile political environment. Hampered by state laws that discouraged and often prohibited their development, proprietary hospitals, when their existence was permitted at all, were tolerated because they filled a gap caused by the shortage of other facilities.[20]

When proprietary hospitals do compete with nonproprietaries, they suffer from some important competitive disadvantages imposed by government policy. First, nonproprietary hospitals are subjected neither to real property taxes nor corporate income taxes because they

18 Charles Phelps, "Public Sector Medicine: History and Analysis," in Cotton Lindsay, ed., *New Directions in Public Health Care: A Prescription for the 1980s* (San Francisco: Institute for Contemporary Studies, 1980), pp. 160–62.

19 Ibid.

20 Herbert Klarman, *The Economics of Health* (New York: Columbia University Press, 1965), p. 113.

are "nonprofit organizations." Proprietary hospitals, on the other hand, pay such taxes on the same basis as any other corporation. A second and more important disadvantage derives from the Hill-Burton Hospital Construction Act of 1946, which provides federal funds for building and equipping public and voluntary *nonprofit* hospitals. Between 1947 and 1966 the Hill-Burton program provided support for the construction of 1,680 new hospitals and 2,998 additions and alterations to existing hospitals.[21]

A third disadvantage stems from the federal government's policy on charitable contributions: Contributions to nonprofit hospitals are tax-deductible; contributions to proprietary hospitals are not. To understand how important this provision of the tax law is, consider the fact that from 1960 to 1966 between 26 percent and 34 percent of all funds for hospital expansion came from philanthropic sources.[22] Nonprofit hospitals also receive a considerable amount of charitable support that goes directly toward underwriting current operating expenses.[23]

Relative to proprietary hospitals, then, nonprofit hospitals escape the burdens of property taxes and income taxes; finance much of their capital equipment and facilities through government funds; and cover many of their current and capital expenses through private charitable contributions that are generally not available to proprietaries because of provisions in the federal income-tax law. In many states they enjoy competitive advantages as a result of a series of court rulings and legislative acts.

These advantages generally stem from the traditional rule prohibiting the "corporate" practice of medicine. The following is a typical statement of the rule and its rationale:

> While a corporation is in some sense a person, and for many purposes is so considered, yet, as regards the learned professions which can only be practiced by persons who have received a license to do so after an examination as to their knowledge of the subject, it is recognized that a corporation cannot be licensed to practice such a profession.[24]

21U.S. Department of Health, Education and Welfare, *Hill-Burton Program Progress Report, July 1, 1947, June 30, 1966* (Washington, D.C.: U.S. Government Printing Office), p. 32.

22Dorothy Rice and Barbara Cooper, "National Health Expenditures, 1950–66," *Social Security Bulletin* 31 (April 1968): 3–22.

23Cotton Lindsay and James Buchanan, "The Organization and Financing of Medical Care in the United States," in British Medical Association, *Health Services Financing* (London: British Medical Association, 1970), p. 548.

24Alanson W. Willcox, "Hospitals and the Corporate Practice of Medicine," *Cornell*

Some courts have applied this rule to proprietary corporations but not to nonprofit corporations.[25] State legislatures have written such distinctions into law. In New York, for example, proprietary hospitals may be operated by single owners or by partnerships, but not by corporations.[26] No such restriction is imposed on nonprofit hospitals.

Often the proscription on the corporate practice of medicine means that the hospital managers may not interfere in the professional decisions of the resident physicians. In some cases it has meant that the hospital cannot collect fees from patients for physicians' services. In other instances, it has meant that physicians may not be employed by nonphysicians.[27] Even when these rules apply equally to profit and nonprofit institutions, the proprietary hospital remains at a disadvantage. Whether the proprietaries can exist in the face of these competitive disadvantages is doubtful unless they are allowed to act innovatively, to try new methods and techniques for reducing costs and improving efficiency.

Innovative activity, however, is precisely what the courts and the legislatures have sought to discourage. The effect of most legal restrictions is to compel private hospitals to fit into the mold set by the voluntaries. Consider the case of *Manlove* v. *Wilmington General Hospital.*[28] In this case the court ruled that a private hospital that maintains an emergency room is required to render services when it reasonably determines that an emergency exists. Ironically, it was the hospital, not the doctors who practice in it, that was required to make the service available.

One of the unfortunate consequences of the Hill-Burton Act was that it required states to license hospitals as a condition for receiving federal funds. By 1975 almost every state had adopted hospital and nursing home licensure laws administered by state agencies.[29] Such agencies can be, and apparently are, used to stifle the development of proprietary hospitals and limit their ability to compete with nonproprietaries.[30]

Law Quarterly 45 (1960): 438. See also, Horace Hansen, "Group Health Plans - A Twenty-Year Legal Review," *Minnesota Law Review* 42 (1958): 527-48.

[25]Forgotson, Roemer, and Newman, p. 403.

[26]Steinwald and Neuhauser, p. 835.

[27]Forgotson, Roemer, and Newman, pp. 402-3.

[28]53 Delaware 338, 169 A.2d 18 (1961).

[29]See Philip Kissam, "Physicians Assistant and Nurse Practitioner Laws: A Study of Health Law Reform," *Kansas Law Review* 24 (1975): 53.

[30]Berry, p. 835. See also David Salkever, "Competition Among Hospitals," in Warren

TABLE 4.3

Market Shares for Hospital Admissions and Outpatient Visits (in Percentages)

Year	Type of Hospital					
	Proprietary		*Voluntary*		*State and Local Government*	
	Admissions	OPV	Admissions	OPV	Admissions	OPV
1960	7	—	73	—	20	—
1965	7	4	72	65	21	31
1970	7	4	72	68	21	28
1978	8	4	71	68	21	28

SOURCE: Derived from American Hospital Association, *American Hospital Association Guide to the Health Care Field: 1979 Edition* (Chicago: American Hospital Association, 1979), table 1.

Two examples of how regulatory authority can be used to discriminate against proprietary hospitals are furnished by New York City. In 1964 the city's hospital code was revised to limit the practice of surgery in proprietary hospitals to board-certified surgeons. In a test case in which the law was upheld, a court ruled that a general practitioner could not continue practicing surgery in proprietary hospitals despite the fact that he had done so for many years and that there was no apparent indication that he was unqualified to continue doing so.[31] In a more dramatic case in 1976, the mayor of New York City attempted to exercise his authority by forcing the outright closure of nine proprietary hospitals operating in the city.[32]

In spite of the competitive disadvantages and the hostile treatment they have received from courts, state legislatures, and planning agencies, proprietary hospitals have survived remarkably well, as is apparent from the statistics presented in table 4.3. For more than a decade proprietary hospitals have maintained a fairly stable share of the market for hospital admissions and for outpatient visits.

Bruce Steinwald and Duncan Neuhauser have completed a detailed

Greenberg, ed., *Competition in the Health Care Sector: Past, Present and Future* (Germantown, Md.: Aspen Systems Corporation, 1978), pp. 150–51.

31See Alonzo Yerby, "Regulation of Health Manpower," in National Academy of Sciences, *Controls on Health Care: Papers of the Conference on Regulation in the Health Industry*, January 7–9, 1974 (Washington, D.C.: National Academy of Sciences, 1975), p. 96.

32"Radical Surgery," *Wall Street Journal*, 27 January 1976.

study of the history of proprietary hospitals in the United States.[33] Their principal finding was that proprietary hospitals have historically prospered in areas where the demand for hospital services outstripped the supply of services provided by nonprofit hospitals. As soon as the marketplace for hospital services began to stabilize, however, proprietary hospitals tended to leave the market, often simply by converting to nonprofit status. The fact that proprietary hospitals tend to enter and exit the market fairly rapidly helps explain why they typically are small in size and low in capital costs.

It is not known precisely why government policies that inhibit the growth and survival of proprietary hospitals developed, or what role was played by organized medicine. A number of health economists have pointed out, however, that professional opinion has traditionally been biased against the proprietaries.[34] Duncan Neuhauser gives the following explanation for this prejudice:

> The professional ideology assumes that the professional is an expert as a result of his years of education and learning. Since he knows more about his area he should tell others what they "need." Consistent with this is the idea that the public is unwise and unknowing. This is in contrast to the idea of consumer sovereignty where the consumer is the best judge of his own desires. Physicians have tended toward the former ideology and businessmen and economists toward the latter. But in the last analysis, until the day comes when we can plant electrodes in peoples' skulls to measure utilities, this must remain an ideological assumption.[35]

Implicit in Neuhauser's explanation is the idea that proprietary hospitals are more likely to cater to the demands of the consumer, whereas nonprofit hospitals are more likely to cater to the interests of the "experts." But there is another reason why professional opinion tends to be prejudiced against proprietary hospitals, and this reason is wholly financial.

AMA Controls in the Hospital Sector

Writing in *Harper's* over thirty years ago, Milton Mayer argued the American Medical Association has "life and death" powers over the

[33]Steinwald and Neuhauser, pp. 817–38.

[34]See, for example, Lindsay and Buchanan, p. 548; Steinwald and Neuhauser, p. 835; and Duncan Neuhauser, "The Future of Proprietaries in American Health Services," in Clark Havighurst, ed., *Regulating Health Facilities Construction: Proceedings of a Conference on Health Planning, Certificates of Need, and Market Entry* (Washington, D.C.: American Enterprise Institute for Public Policy Research, 1974), p. 241.

[35]Neuhauser, p. 239.

nation's hospitals, similar to the control it asserts over the nation's medical schools.[36] In 1958 Reuben Kessel echoed this charge.[37] To understand the source of the AMA's power, it is necessary to turn first to hospital intern and residency programs.

In marked contrast to the facilities available for pre-MD training in the United States, there are a plethora of facilities for post-MD training.[38] Between 1940 and 1960 the number of approved residencies in hospitals increased 600 percent, while the output of medical graduates rose only 35 percent.[39] Moreover, the growth of supply has been outstripping the growth of demand. In the 1960s, for example, 20 percent of all approved internships and residencies in the United States were unfilled, despite the fact that foreign-trained physicians occupied one-third of these positions.[40]

Why is it that the facilities for post-MD training are so disproportionately large, relative to the facilities for pre-MD training? The reason is that hospitals, and the physicians who practice in them, derive an economic benefit from post-MD training programs, whereas they derive no comparable benefit from pre-MD programs. Kessel has explained the benefit:

> Hospitals value highly participation in internship and residency training programs. These programs are valued highly because at the prevailing wage for intern services, it is possible to produce hospital care more cheaply with interns than without them. Interns to hospitals are like coke to the steel industry: in both cases, it is perfectly possible to produce the final product without these raw materials; in both cases, the final product can be produced more cheaply by using these particular raw materials.[41]

By contrast, first- and second-year medical students have proved to be of little value to hospitals. Third- and fourth-year are of some

[36]Milton S. Mayer, "The Dogged Retreat of the Doctors," *Harper's*, December 1949, p. 27.

[37]Reuben Kessel, "Price Discrimination in Medicine," *Journal of Law and Economics* 1 (October 1958): 20–53.

[38]Kessel has observed the double irony in the current structure of medical education: The more advanced the training, the greater is the availability of facilities, and this more specialized and advanced training often takes place outside of medical schools. See Reuben Kessel, "The AMA and the Supply of Physicians," *Law and Contemporary Problems*, Spring 1970, p. 277.

[39]Richard Shryock, *Medical Licensing in America: 1650–1965* (Baltimore: Johns Hopkins University Press, 1967), p. 91.

[40]See Public Health Service, *Health Manpower Sourcebook*, 1968, table 28.

[41]Kessel, "Price Discrimination in Medicine," p. 30.

value, but they are not worth as much as post-MD students.[42] In any event, as we have seen, additional pre-MD students would expand the supply of physicians. The discrepancy between the availability of these two types of training programs, then, is consistent with the overall desire of organized medicine to maximize physicians' incomes.

How does a hospital go about establishing internship and residency programs? It turns to the AMA. In most states internship is a necessary condition for physician licensure. Although the training is done by the hospitals themselves, these hospitals must receive "class A" ratings from the AMA's Council on Medical Education. The approval of hospital internship programs is technically the responsibility of state licensing boards, but the lists of approved schools are generally identical to the AMA Council's list.[43] In a similar way, the AMA also "approves" residency programs.[44]

The revocation of a class A rating is probably not a fear of large, renowned teaching hospitals, but for hospitals in a more vulnerable position, loss of this rating would mean loss of residents and interns, and, as a consequence, higher production costs of hospital services. Since most nonproprietary hospitals in this country are approved for at least intern training, the AMA's power of approval is a potential threat to a great many hospitals.[45]

Kessel has argued that this control over hospitals by the AMA has been used to induce them to abide by the Mundt Resolution, which advises "approved" hospitals that their staff ought to be composed solely of members of local medical societies.[46] As a result, membership in these societies is of enormous importance to practicing physicians. Lack of membership means that the physician cannot join a hospital staff.

In most hospitals today the doctors themselves have de facto control over staff appointments. In general, the hospitals' lay trustees simply act as a rubber stamp for the medical staff in matters of staff privileges.[47] This fact, coupled with the great internal solidarity and

[42]Kessel, "The AMA and the Supply of Physicians," p. 277.

[43]Elton Rayack, "Restrictive Practices of Organized Medicine," *The Antitrust Bulletin*, 1968, pp. 664-65.

[44]Kessel, "Price Discrimination in Medicine," pp. 29-30.

[45]Ibid.

[46]David R. Hyde, Payson Wolff, Anne Gross, and Elliott Lee Hoffman, "The American Medical Association: Power, Purpose and Politics in Organized Medicine," *Yale Law Journal* 63 (May 1954): p. 952.

[47]Rayack, pp. 708-9.

cohesion that has traditionally existed in the medical community, means that hospital doctors and local medical societies often see eye-to-eye on the value of using their power to promote the goals of organized medicine.

Kessel has explained what all of this means to the ordinary physician whose inclination would be to pursue his own financial self-interest:

> For doctors dependent upon hospitals in order to carry out their practice, and presumably this constitutes the bulk of the profession, being cut off from access to hospitals constitutes a partial revocation of their license to practice medicine.... More significantly, doctors are subject to very severe losses indeed if they should be expelled from their local county medical associations or be refused admission to membership. It is this weapon, expulsion from county medical associations, that is probably the most formidable sanction employed to keep doctors from maximizing their personal incomes by cutting prices to high income patients. "Unethical" doctors, i.e., price cutters, can be in large part removed as a threat to the structure of prices that discriminates in terms of income by the use of this weapon. For potential unethical physicians, it pays not to cut prices if cutting prices means being cut off from hospitals.[48]

Loss of hospital privileges is not the only penalty suffered by physicians who are expelled from, or who lose membership in, local medical societies. Membership in a county medical society is generally a necessary condition for admission to a number of specialty board examinations, and passing these examinations is a necessary condition for specialty ratings.[49] Obviously membership in a county medical society has nothing to do with a candidate's qualifications for specialty ratings, but this provision represents an important form of control over newcomers to the profession. Young physicians tend to aspire to specialty board ratings, and they are also the physicians most likely to be price cutters.[50]

Nonmembers of county medical societies may also find it very costly, or even impossible, to purchase malpractice insurance. In the 1950s insurance rates were sometimes 20 to 100 percent higher for nonmembers, and some insurance companies refused to issue them policies.[51] One reason for this phenomenon may be that county societies play a

[48]Kessel, "Price Discrimination in Medicine," p. 31.

[49]Hyde and Wolff, pp. 938, 952.

[50]Kessel, "Price Discrimination in Medicine," p. 32.

[51]Hyde and Wolff, p. 951.

crucial role in protecting their members against malpractice suits. According to Kessel they serve as judge and jury for an accused colleague before the case goes to court. If his fellow members find him innocent, they will be available to act as expert witnesses in his behalf.[52] As a consequence, the position of a plaintiff in a malpractice suit is much stronger if the defendant is a nonmember than if he is a member.

Physicians who do not belong to county medical societies may suffer in other ways. They may receive no referrals from other physicians or lose the opportunity to engage in consultations with them. They may even be completely ostracized by the medical community. One writer has described the importance of these sanctions in the following way:

> First, of course, and never out of use, is social pressure in a small group. The social life of the county society is important to some doctors. Few can wholly disregard it, simply because a doctor can ill afford more than a few enemies, certainly not the hostility of an organized group in positions of local prominence. His reputation is a fragile thing, and his income and practice depend upon being called in consultation, though perhaps more vitally on being able to call his colleagues in emergencies. Ostracism becomes a terrible weapon in such a business.[53]

Organized medicine has used or threatened to use the power to expel physicians from county medical societies on numerous occasions in the pursuit of its objectives: to discourage price cutting, advertising, engaging in prepayment insurance plans, and even testifying in malpractice suits.[54] That the principal purpose of this sanction is to protect physicians' incomes rather than the public's health is demonstrated by some of the more ludicrous rules that are enforced. Making specialty board ratings conditional on membership in a medical society is one example. Another is the fact that all newcomers are made probationary members when they join some medical societies, even if they were former presidents of county societies elsewhere.[55] Newcomers are a group whose members are trying to acquire a practice

[52] Kessel, "Price Discrimination in Medicine," p. 44.

[53] Oliver Garceau, *The Political Life of the American Medical Association* (Cambridge, Mass: Harvard University Press, 1941), p. 103.

[54] Examples of the use of this power to thwart disapproved insurance schemes will be presented in chapter 5. Examples of the use of this power to thwart the other three activities were presented in chapter 3.

[55] Hyde and Wolff, p. 941, n. 20 and p. 951, n. 83.

and, therefore, much more likely to be price cutters than physicians with an established practice.[56]

There is also evidence that internships and residencies are designed largely for the benefit of practicing physicians and hospitals rather than for the pursuit of any social purpose. The report on graduate medical education (Millis Report), for example, suggests that the internship no longer performs any educative function and that the length of residencies is related more to the desires for house staff than to educational considerations.[57]

Finally, organized medicine has not only maintained a hostile attitude toward hospitals that threaten the continued exercise of its power over the practice of medicine by physicians — e.g., proprietary hospitals — but has also taken steps to combat group medical practices that will conceivably compete with hospitals. In 1978, for example, the *New York Times* reported the following cases in which group practices ran afoul of the AMA's rule against "mixed" corporate medicine:

- A West Virginia rheumatologist was enjoined from working with a paraprofessional physician's assistant.
- A Texas orthopedic surgeon was unable to practice with a physical therapist.
- A Michigan psychiatrist was criticized for sharing clients with a social worker and a psychologist.[58]

As we noted in chapter 2, many, if not most, of the practices we have described here are now illegal, or probably illegal, as a result of recent court rulings and a ruling by a Federal Trade Commission judge. Nonetheless, the legacy of over seventy years of AMA domination of the medical marketplace is a strong one.

The Economic Effects of AMA Policies

Among the more pronounced economic effects of AMA policies on hospitals are the following:

A greater degree of price discrimination among specialists than among general practitioners. The AMA clearly has more powerful

[56]See G. Stocking and M. Watkins, *Monopoly and Free Enterprise* (New York: Twentieth-Century Fund, 1951), p. 117; and Kessel, "Price Discrimination in Medicine," p. 43.

[57]Citizens Commission on Graduate Education, *The Graduate Education of Physicians* (1966), pp. 23, 58.

[58]"The AMA's Bad Case," *New York Times*, 6 December 1978.

weapons to discipline doctors who practice in hospitals than it does to discipline doctors who do not. Moreover, in conjunction with the growth of this power came an increased interest in new areas of "unethical" practice, such as fee-splitting. In general, fee-splitting allows young specialists to compete for referrals from general practitioners and other doctors. The rule against fee-splitting, therefore, serves to protect the established specialists against competition from their younger rivals.[59]

As a consequence, the AMA has been far more effective in protecting systematic price discrimination in the market for the services of specialists than it has been in the market for the services of general practitioners. This has been particularly true in the surgical specialties:

> The presence of systematic price discrimination in the provision of surgical services is evidence of the absence of price competition made possible by organized medicine's control over access to hospital beds. Comparable control over fees for office visits does not exist, and consumer knowledge of the prices for office visits is considerably greater.[60]

How much price discrimination exists in the surgical specialties? According to Kessel, it is not unknown for patients to be charged surgical fees that are as much as 50 percent higher than the Medicare rate, although the Medicare rate is supposed to reflect the prevailing price in the community.[61]

Excessive specialization among physicians. The fact that the restrictive practices of organized medicine have been more successful in markets for the services of specialists than in markets for the services of nonspecialists has meant that average incomes of specialists are artificially high relative to the incomes of nonspecialists. This may be one of the contributing factors in the rapid increase in specialization among physicians over the last two decades. Table 4.4 compares the earnings of general practitioners with the earnings of other practitioners and male college graduates from 1947 to 1975. As the table shows, but for the impact of Medicare and Medicaid, introduced in 1965, the ratio of GP earnings to the earnings of college graduates has remained fairly constant. The ratio in 1975 stood at 2.48 — exactly what it was in 1959. The behavior of the ratio of GP earnings to the

[59]Kessel, "Price Discrimination in Medicine," p. 52, n. 95.

[60]Kessel, "The AMA and the Supply of Physicians," p. 280.

[61]Ibid., p. 281.

TABLE 4.4

Earnings Ratio of GPs to All Physicians and to Males with 4 Years of College

Year	GPs to All Physicians	GPs to Males with 4 Years of College	Year	GPs to All Physicians	GPs to Males with 4 Years of College
1947	.925	1.92	1967	.903	2.88
1951	.925	2.18	1968	—	2.75
1955	.925	2.42	1969	—	2.71
1959	.905	2.48	1970	.862	2.79
1961	—	2.59	1971	—	2.72
1962	.893	2.58	1972	.808	2.54
1963	.888	2.54	1973	.800	2.62
1964	.861	2.70	1974	.753	2.51
1965	.866	2.69	1975	.742	2.48
1966	.861	2.76	1976	.752	—

SOURCE: Keith Leffler, *Explanations in Search of Facts: A Critique of "A Study of Physicians' Fees"* (Coral Gables, Florida: Law and Economics Center, University of Miami School of Law, 1978), table 2. Reprinted by permission.

earnings of specialists, however, tells a different story. Whereas average GP incomes in 1947 were 92.5 percent of the average incomes of specialists, by 1975 they had fallen to 75.2 percent.

Young physicians have apparently responded to these incentives by entering specialized practice in increasing numbers. From 1949 to 1975 the percentage of physicians who practiced general medicine fell from 63.5 percent to 17.2 percent, while the percentage of physicians who specialized rose from 36.5 percent to 82.8 percent.[62] Moreover, among the particular specialties it appears that hospital-based specialties are attracting more young physicians than specialties that are not hospital-based. Unfilled vacancies in the surgical specialties, for example, are generally smaller than unfilled vacancies in the nonsurgical specialties.[63]

Artificially high prices for surgical procedures. It might seem that

[62]Keith Leffler, *Explanations in Search of Facts: A Critique of 'A Study of Physicians Fees'* (Coral Gables, Fla.: Law and Economics Center, University of Miami School of Law, 1978), Preface.

[63]American Medical Association, *Directory of Approved Internships and Residencies, 1968-69* (Chicago: American Medical Association, 1969), pp. 8-9. The overall percentage filled is 81%. For thoracic surgery it is 91%; plastic surgery, 87%; colon and rectal surgery, 92% and neurologic surgery, 91%. By contrast, the percentage filled in general practice is 48%; pathology, 58%; and psychiatry, 76%.

increased entry into the medical specialties would tend to reduce the average fees charged in these specialties. As it turns out, however, specialists have become increasingly zealous in protecting their domain against invasion by nonspecialists. Precisely because they have more to gain from such involvement, specialists tend to be overrepresented in the AMA hierarchy.[64] Moreover, among the specialists themselves, surgeons tend to be especially overrepresented in medical politics. As one observer notes, "Our medical societies are not merely specialist dominated; they are surgeon dominated."[65]

Involvement in medical politics apparently pays off in conflicts over staff privileges. For example, it is apparently not uncommon for surgeons to attempt to prevent general practitioners from performing surgery in hospitals.[66] Where they have succeeded in doing so, income differentials between the two groups have tended to widen. Elton Rayack recently compared physicians' earnings in the eastern United States with those in the West.[67] In both parts of the country the ratio of GPs to specialists is about the same. Medical staff restrictionism is apparently more common in the East, however, and the income statistics reflect this. In the West the 1959 median income of specialists was only 9 percent greater than the income of general practitioners. That same year, in the more restrictionist East, the specialists' median income exceeded the general practitioners' by 22 percent.[68]

Isn't it better for a patient to use a specialist rather than a general practitioner? Not necessarily. Specialty restrictionism tends to raise the fees patients pay and to cause wasteful use of resources as well. Elton Rayack explains why:

> To the extent that specialty restrictionism has led to the use of the higher-priced services of the specialist as a substitute for the general practitioners' services, *on the assumption that the G.P. could have provided services of equal quality,* there is definitely a malallocation of resources. The loss is not simply in terms of the higher prices paid by the consumers of medical services: even more significant is the waste of resources involved in training specialists when the smaller amount of resources devoted to the training of general practitioners

64Kessel, "Price Discrimination in Medicine," p. 43.

65Herbert Berger, "Are Surgical Fees Too High?" *Medical Economics* 32 (June 1955): 272.

66Rayack, p. 709.

67Ibid., p. 715.

68See *Physicians' Earning and Expenses* (Oradell, N.J.: Medical Economics, Inc., 1960), p. 12.

> would have been adequate. If a patient has a brain tumor, it is obvious that it would be more desirable for him to be operated on by a neurosurgeon than by a general practitioner. However, most common ailments, normal delivery of babies, minor surgery, and even uncomplicated major surgery can surely be handled by general practitioners; in these cases, to compel the use of costly services of specialists is to waste resources.[69]

Other inefficiencies in the production of hospital services. Perhaps the most serious economic effect of AMA policies is the absence of price competition among the hospitals. Numerous observers have noted that instead of competing on the basis of price, hospitals tend to compete on the basis of the availability and sophistication of services and facilities.[70] Moreover, competition is often, if not usually, competition for members of the medical staff rather than competition for patients. Once the hospital obtains the patronage of the physician, it expects the patronage of his patients to follow. The hospital may even demand it. Some hospitals apparently require that staff physicians send a substantial portion of their hospitalized patients as a condition of active staff membership.[71]

The result is a wasteful and inefficient hospital sector. Not only do numerous hospitals provide services and facilities that are grossly uneconomical, but the harmful effects on patients extend well beyond their pocketbooks. As an example, Professors Herman and Anne Somers cite a presidential commission for the following rather astonishing statistics:

> . . . 30% of the 777 hospitals equipped to do closed-heart surgery had no such case in the year under study. Of the 548 hospitals that had cases, 87% did fewer than one operation per week. Of all hospitals equipped to do open-heart surgery, 77% did not average even one operation per week, and 41% averaged under one per month. Little of this work was of an emergency nature, and *the mortality rate for both procedures is "far higher . . . than in institutions with a full work load."*[72]

[69]Rayack, p. 713. For similar views, see Herbert Ratner, "Deficiencies in Present Day Medical Education," *GP* (July 1965): 187.

[70]See, for example, Salkever, p. 201.

[71]See the case studies described in Milton Roemer and Jay Friedman, *Doctors in Hospitals: Medical Staff Organization and Hospital Performance* (Baltimore: Johns Hopkins University Press, 1971).

[72]Herman and Anne Somers, *Medicare and the Hospitals* (Washington, D.C.: The Brookings Institution, 1967), p. 198. Emphasis added.

V. CONTROLS ON THE METHOD OF PAYMENT: MEDICAL INSURANCE

Our orthodox medical brethren ... adopt the fiercely partisan attitude of a powerful trade union; they demand legislation against the competition of "scabs."

William James, 1898

Medical insurance in one form or another has existed in the United States for almost a century. As early as the 1880s prepayment plans for hospital expenses and industrial medical care plans were in operation. Surgical benefits in individual insurance policies appeared as early as 1903, and medical benefits were included in individual policies by 1910.[1] During the next decade health insurance even became a political issue: In the presidential campaign of 1912, the Progressive party, under Theodore Roosevelt, adopted compulsory national health insurance as one of the planks in its platform.[2]

The attitude of the American Medical Association toward medical insurance has gone through several cycles. Prior to 1920 the AMA, through editorials in the *Journal of the American Medical Association*, supported national health insurance. By the 1930s the organization had come full swing and openly opposed even voluntary medical insurance. In the late 1930s, however, the AMA settled on a policy course that it has pursued to this day: Medical insurance schemes are approved by the AMA so long as they are either directly or indirectly controlled by organized medicine.[3]

AMA Policies Toward Medical Insurance

There are two basic types of medical insurance.[4] Under cash indemnity medical insurance, doctors and patients determine medical fees jointly at the time the medical services are sold, just as if there were no

[1] O. D. Dickerson, *Health Insurance* (Homewood, Ill.: Richard D. Irwin, 1963), pp. 151, 173.

[2] Henry Steele Commager, ed., *Documents of American History*, 3rd ed. (New York: F. S. Crafts & Co., 1947), p. 255.

[3] Elton Rayack, *Professional Power and American Medicine: The Economics of the American Medical Association* (Cleveland: World Publishing Co., 1967), chapter 5.

[4] For a detailed analysis of a wide variety of insurance plans and their economic effects,

medical insurance. All or part of the medical bill is then paid by the insurance plan, depending on the specifics of the policy. Examples of medical indemnity insurance are Blue Cross and Blue Shield plans.

Nonindemnity medical insurance plans, on the other hand, provide medical care itself rather than the funds with which to buy those services. Such plans are often called prepaid plans because the patient's insurance premiums generally cover all of the medical services he subsequently consumes. Examples of such plans are health maintenance organizations (HMOs).

These two types of plans differ enormously in their economic effects on the providers of medical insurance. If insurance companies are not too aggressive in monitoring fees, indemnity insurance does little more than increase the ability of patients to pay their medical bills. Generally speaking, patients are free to select the physician and hospital of their choice, and physicians are free to set their fees as they like, including the all-important freedom to price discriminate.

Nonindemnity insurance, on the other hand, generally restricts the patient to a select group of physicians and medical facilities. Cost of membership in such plans typically varies according to age, family size, scope of coverage, quality of service, etc. But premiums are generally independent of income, which means that such plans do not engage in price discrimination against high-income groups.[5]

Indemnity insurance tends to benefit the entire medical community by increasing the overall demand for medical care and leaving practitioners free to engage in monopolistic pricing practices. Nonindemnity, prepaid plans, on the other hand, tend to benefit only the group of providers associated with the plan, often at the expense of all other competing providers. Moreover, since prepaid plans typically set premiums that are independent of income, they potentially represent a means for cutting prices to high-income patients.

The economic principles governing these two types of medical insurance plans help explain why patients have often found nonindemnity insurance plans attractive in a market dominated by the noncompetitive pricing policies of organized medicine. They also help explain why the AMA has so vigorously opposed nonindemnity insurance. The AMA has not merely condemned prepaid insurance

---

see H. E. Frech III and Paul B. Ginsburg, *Public Insurance in Private Medical Markets: Some Problems of National Health Insurance* (Washington, D.C.: American Enterprise Institute for Public Policy Research, 1978).

[5]Reuben Kessel, "Price Discrimination in Medicine," *Journal of Law and Economics* 1 (October 1958): 33.

schemes, it has gone so far as to denounce them as unethical. According to an AMA House of Delegates resolution adopted in 1932, such plans are "unethical":

> 1. Where there is solicitation of patients, either directly or indirectly
>
> 2. Where there is competition and underbidding to secure the contract
>
> 3. When the compensation is inadequate to secure good medical service
>
> 4. When there is interference with reasonable competition in a community
>
> 5. When free choice of physicians is prevented
>
> 6. When the contract because of any of its provisions is contrary to sound public policy[6]

Note that five of the six criteria for determining whether a prepaid plan is unethical are obviously intended to protect the economic position of other physicians. The sixth is open-ended, making it possible to condemn any form of prepaid practice. As Elton Rayack has written, "Clearly what was involved [in the list of conditions] was a question of medical economics rather than medical ethics, though the two are often synonymous in the jargon of organized medicine."[7]

Some Case Histories

Organized medicine has gone to great lengths to ensure that unethical prepaid plans do not flourish in the market for medical insurance. Just how far it has gone is vividly illustrated by a number of dramatic battles in which prepaid plans struggled to survive the destructive efforts of organized medicine. Below is a brief summary of some of the most important cases.[8]

[6]Listed in Rayack, *Professional Power and American Medicine*, p. 152. These conditions were contained in a minority report to the report of the committee on the Costs of Medical Care. See *Medical Care for the American People*, Report of the Committee on the Costs of Medical Care (Chicago: University of Chicago Press, 1932). The minority report was subsequently endorsed by the AMA House of Delegates in 1932. See American Medical Association, *Digest of Official Actions*, 1846–1958 (Chicago: AMA, 1959), p. 314.

[7]Rayack, p. 153.

[8]Convenient summaries of the facts in these cases may be found in Kessel, pp. 34–41; and/or Rayack, pp. 180–195.

Farmers Union Hospital Association In 1929 Dr. Michael Shadid founded in Elk City, Oklahoma, what was perhaps the first consumer cooperative in the field of medical care, the Farmers Union Hospital Association. Members of the cooperative owned their hospital, paid staff doctors a fixed salary, and received medical care on a prepaid basis. From its inception and for more than two decades the cooperative was harassed by the Beckham County Medical Society.

The prime target was Shadid himself. He was expelled from the local medical society in an ingenious way. Since Shadid had been a respected member of the local medical society for twenty years, there was no legitimate reason for expulsion, so the society dissolved for six months and then reorganized, apparently for the sole purpose of not inviting Shadid to become a member. For more than two decades other members of the hospital association were also barred from local medical society membership.

Loss of hospital privileges was not a serious blow to Shadid's organization because the group had its own hospital. Other tactics were more effective, however. The local medical society was able to prevent doctors who were known to be coming to Oklahoma to join Shadid's organization from getting a license to practice. It was also able to force the departure of a doctor who had been associated with Shadid's organization for a substantial period of time, to keep Shadid out of a two-week postgraduate course at the Cook County School of Medicine (the course was open only to members in good standing of their local medical societies), and to get enough of Shadid's doctors drafted during the war so that the life of the hospital association was endangered.

Shadid was equal to the challenge, however. He was shrewd enough to draw members of the politically powerful Farmers Union into his organization and in the political battle between the farmers and the doctors, the governor of the state sided with the farmers. The hospital association also brought suit against the Beckham County Medical Association and its members, charging conspiracy in restraint of trade. In the eventual out-of-court settlement, the medical association agreed to accept the medical staff of the cooperative as members.[9]

Group Health Association Group Health Association (GHA) of Washington, D.C., was not as fortunate as Farmers Union — it did

[9]The story of Shadid and his organization may be found in M. A. Shadid, *A Doctor for the People* (New York: The Vanguard Press, 1939); and M. A. Shadid, *Doctors of Today and Tomorrow* (New York: Cooperative League of the U.S.A., 1947).

not own its own hospital. Consequently, after its formation in 1937, Group Health found itself dependent on the use of existing hospitals in the community. The first response of the District of Columbia Medical Society was to have the organization declared illegal on the grounds that it was engaged in the "corporate practice of medicine." Failing that, the society expelled or barred from membership all doctors who participated in the Group Health plan. Doctors who consulted with GHA physicians were threatened with expulsion, and all local hospitals were pressured to close their doors to GHA physicians. The case even attracted the attention of the national office of the AMA, which declared GHA "unethical" and sent representatives to advise the local medical society.

Fortunately for GHA, it was located in Washington, D.C., and therefore was under the jurisdiction of federal laws — the Sherman Antitrust Act in particular. In 1943 a unanimous Supreme Court found the AMA and the local medical society guilty of criminal conspiracy under federal antitrust laws. Although the fines were ludicrously low — $2,500 against the AMA and $1,500 against the District of Columbia Medical Society — the ruling made it possible for GHA to flourish in successful competition with fee-for-service medicine.[10]

Group Health Cooperative of Puget Sound The Group Health Cooperative of Puget Sound (GHC) was organized in 1946 in Puget Sound, Washington, by leaders in granges, labor unions, and consumer cooperatives. Soon afterward the King County Medical Association launched a concerted drive to destroy it. Staff members were expelled from the medical association and new additions to the staff were barred from society membership. The medical society also refused to accept transfers of membership from other county medical societies by doctors who were expected to join the cooperative. Although GHC owned its own health clinic, members of its staff were barred from all existing hospitals in the community. Staff members were also barred from many scientific meetings and were unable to consult with orthodox members of the profession.

Despite this harassment GHC survived. The cooperative brought suit against the King County Medical Association, charging that the defendants conspired to drive the cooperative out of business. The

[10]See Committee on Research in Medical Economics, *Restrictions on Free Enterprise in Medicine* (New York: CRFEM, 1949), pp. 12–13; Morris Fishbein, *A History of the American Medical Association* (Philadelphia: W. B. Saunders, 1947), pp. 534–39; and *American Medical Association* v. *United States*, 317 U.S. 519, 536 (1943).

legal victory — this time in state courts — resulted in no award of damages, but the cooperative's physicians did gain access to local hospitals.[11]

Civic Medical Center Like some other prepaid schemes, the Civic Medical Center (CMC) in Chicago did not own its own hospital. In 1946 not one of the fifteen staff members had succeeded in being admitted to the Chicago Medical Society. Appeals to the Illinois State Medical Society and the AMA proved to be fruitless. Even the direct appeal by a committee of patients of CMC to the local medical society was of no avail. As a result, physicians on the staff of the CMC clinic were able to practice in only two hospitals in the entire Chicago area. Moreover, in these two hospitals they were given only limited staff privileges, a restriction that seriously hampered the operations of the clinic. In one of the two hospitals, for example, CMC physicians could not schedule surgery more than two days in advance.

This case is especially interesting because it illustrates how the military draft can be used as a weapon against unorthodox practitioners. During World War II it appears that some of the physicians in the CMC group were disqualified as medical officers in the navy and instead were drafted as enlisted men. Applications to serve as medical officers were rejected by the navy unless accompanied by a letter certifying that the candidate was a member in good standing of his local medical society.[12]

The Ross-Loos Clinic The Ross-Loos plan in Los Angeles is a prepaid plan that began in 1929 and had acquired 127,000 members by 1952. This case is important because it illustrates the AMA's willingness to reach an accommodation with unapproved medical insurance schemes. Initially, the Los Angeles County Medical Association expelled all Ross-Loos doctors from its organization, including a former president of the county medical society. After a series of appeals within the judicial machinery of organized medicine, however, these local actions were reversed.[13]

A possible reason for this reversal is suggested by the testimony of Dr. H. Clifford Loos, a cofounder of Ross-Loos. In response to the question, "Are you handicapped to any extent by the fact that you are

[11]*Group Health, etc.* v. *King County Medical Society,* 39 Washington 2d. 586, 237 P. 2d. 737 (1951).

[12]U.S. Congress, Senate, Committee on Education and Labor, *Hearings on S. 1606, National Health Program,* Part 5, 79th Congress, 2d. Session, pp. 2630 ff.

[13]*Hearings, Health Inquiry,* pp. 1451 ff.

not able to advertise?" Dr. Loos replied, "As far as that goes, we do not care to be big, or bigger. If I had accepted all of the groups who applied to us, we would need our city hall to house us. We have put the brakes on. We can't accept too many. We feel we can't be too big."[14]

As Reuben Kessel has observed, "This constitutes strange behavior indeed for a profit-seeking institution that certainly ought to have no fears of Justice Department action for either being too large or monopolizing an industry."[15] Apparently Ross-Loos reached an understanding with the county medical society that limited its expansion.

The Palo Alto Clinic The Palo Alto Clinic in California is another example of accommodation. The clinic operates a prepaid plan (which does not engage in price discrimination) for the students, faculty, and employees of Stanford University. About 85 percent of the receipts of the Palo Alto Clinic, however, are generated by a fee-for-service practice that lends itself to discriminatory pricing. What explains the extent of prepaid practice by the clinic? According to testimony by the clinic's director, new applications for membership in the prepaid plan are not accepted unless prior approval is obtained from the county medical society.[16] Reuben Kessel explains:

> This suggests that the Palo Alto Clinic is in the position of having to go to its principal competitors for permission to sell its services to new customers. This is comparable to a requirement that a Ford dealer must first obtain the permission of his competing Chevrolet dealer before he can sell Fords to non-Ford owners who have asked for the opportunity to buy them. Probably the county medical society that includes the Palo Alto Clinic does not feel that the present level of sales of prepaid medical services by this clinic is high enough to justify the costs and risks of punitive action.[17]

Legal Restrictions on Medical Insurance Plans

Not only has organized medicine employed a great many professional sanctions to combat the growth of prepaid medical insurance plans, it has also lobbied successfully for legislation that would make such plans illegal. As of 1954, for example, at least twenty states had passed laws designed to prevent prepaid group practice and to keep medical practice on a fee-for-service basis.[18]

14 Ibid., p. 1469.

15 Kessel, p. 40.

16 *Hearings, Health Inquiry*, p. 1559.

17 Kessel, p. 41.

18 *Hearings, Health Inquiry*, p. 1594.

Among the many restrictions faced by would-be prepaid insurance schemes are the class of restrictions included under the prohibition on the "corporate practice of medicine." Among other things, this restriction often means that such plans may be operated only by physicians. In 1950, for example, a survey of state legislation governing medical insurance schemes found that "most of the states [had] restrictive statutes permitting only the medical profession to operate or to control prepayment medical care plans."[19] Moreover, the survey listed as one of the primary objectives of such legislation the desire "to preserve the fee-for-service system as far as possible by controlling the financial administration of the plans."[20]

Another restriction on prepaid schemes is the ban on advertising. Often this prohibition has been applied to prepaid plans but not to indemnity insurance schemes. The professional distinction between these two types of advertising presumably hinges on the fact that indemnity plans are merely selling "insurance," whereas prepaid plans are often selling "medical services" in addition to insurance. The economic distinction, as we have noted, is possibly more important. Indemnity insurance tends to benefit all practicing physicians, whereas prepaid plans benefit only those physicians associated with the plans.[21]

State insurance regulations may also discriminate against nonindemnity insurance schemes. A number of states, for example, require prepaid schemes to maintain large financial reserves, to charge unreasonably low insurance rates, and to limit asset holdings.[22] In general such restrictions are the same as those applied to indemnity insurance, even though prepaid plans do not face the problems these restrictions were designed to address. Prepaid plans, for example, promise benefits in kind, rather than in cash, and hence they do not need to accumulate cash reserves. Moreover, since prepaid plans typically have no deductibles or copayment features, they generally need to charge higher premiums to provide medical services than indemnity plans need to charge for covering those services.

Recent "certificate-of-need" legislation has also hampered the

[19]Horace R. Hansen, "Laws Affecting Group Health Plans," *Iowa Law Review* 35 (1950): 209, 225.

[20]Ibid., p. 209.

[21]See the discussion in Kessel, p. 43.

[22]Frank Sloan and Roger Feldman, "Competition Among Physicians," in Warren Greenberg, ed., *Competition in the Health Care Sector: Past, Present, and Future* (Germantown, Md.: Aspen Systems Corporation, 1978), p. 104.

growth of prepaid medical insurance. These laws usually exempt fee-for-service physicians as noninstitutional providers. Prepaid group practices, however, are considered institutional providers, and as such they must often seek government approval for such items as physicians' office space and major equipment.[23] Certificate-of-need controls may also be used to bar entry to providers whom the medical establishment regards as "undesirable."[24]

State restrictions on medical insurance may have been particularly significant in retarding the growth of Health Maintenance Organizations (HMOs).[25] Loosely defined, an HMO is an organization that accepts contractual responsibility to assure the delivery of a stated range of medical services in exchange for a fixed fee. HMOs are thought to be particularly significant today because they represent the best alternative to indemnity insurance under current market conditions. Recent federal legislation has overridden many restrictive state laws that discriminate against HMOs. We will examine the specifics of this legislation in chapter 7.

Competition and Monopoly in the Market for Medical Insurance

The fact that the AMA prefers indemnity insurance to prepaid group practice does not mean that indemnity insurance poses no threat to the pricing practices of organized medicine.[26] In principle, insurance companies can carefully monitor the services rendered and act

[23]Ibid.

[24]See David Salkever and Thomas Bice, "The Impact of Certificate of Need Controls on Hospital Investment," *Health and Society*, Spring 1976, p. 189.

[25]See Ira Greenberg and Michael Rodburg, "The Role of Prepaid Group Practice in Relieving the Medical Care Crisis," *Harvard Law Review* 84 (February 1971): 887–1001; Robert Holly and Rick Carlson, "The Legal Context for the Development of Health Maintenance Organizations," *Stanford Law Review* 24 (April 1972): 644–86; Institute of Medicine, *Health Maintenance Organizations: Towards a Fair Market Test* (Washington, D.C.: National Academy of Sciences, 1974); and Esther Uyehara and Margaret Thomas, *Health Maintenance Organizations and the HMO Act of 1973* (Santa Monica, Calif., 1975). For the view that most state regulations have not been a serious impediment to the growth of HMOs, see Richard McNeil and Robert Schlenker, "HMOs, Competition, and Government," *Health and Society* (Spring 1975): 195–224.

[26]This section is based largely on Lawrence Goldberg and Warren Greenberg, "The Emergence of Physician-Sponsored Health Insurance: A Historical Perspective," in Warren Greenberg, ed., *Competition in the Health Sector*, pp. 288–321; and Lawrence Goldberg and Warren Greenberg, "The Effect of Physician-Controlled Health Insurance: '*U.S.* v. *Oregon State Medical Society*'", *Journal of Health Politics, Policy and Law* 2 (Spring 1977): 48–78.

aggressively to contain costs. As a recent study of the problem of insurance observes:

> Economic theory suggests and experience confirms that the injection of insurance into a marketplace need not result in uncontrolled cost escalation. Automobile insurers, for example, control the cost of collision-damage claims by requiring multiple estimates or by directly inspecting damage prior to repair. Workmen's compensation insurers conduct safety inspections and use experience-rated premiums to stimulate accident prevention. Manufacturers offering warranties covering repairs by independent dealers have developed a variety of techniques to prevent abuse. In each case, competitive pressure to provide essential protection at the lowest possible price induces cost-cutting actions which are both acceptable to insureds and effective enough to warrant incurring the administrative costs involved.[27]

Dental health insurance is another example. A number of insurance companies actively monitor claims from dentists before authorizing payment for treatment expected to exceed $100. Aetna Life and Casualty's United Automobile Worker's plan is an example. Among the techniques used by Aetna to investigate questionable claims are (1) discussions with the attending dentist; (2) examination of dental X-rays; and (3) case review by Aetna's dental consultant when professional judgment is required.[28]

In medical insurance, however, very little effort appears to be made to control costs. Data from Blue Shield suggest that only 0.04 percent of all benefit claims paid to physicians are disallowed because of questionable practices. Why is medical insurance such a glaring exception to the general pattern in the insurance business? A recent investigation into the historical development of medical insurance in the state of Oregon by Lawrence Goldberg and Warren Greenberg gives some insight into why the market for medical insurance developed as it did.[29]

In the early part of this century, prepaid medical insurance developed both in Oregon and in Washington largely as a result of the hazardous working conditions in the lumber, railroad, and mining industries. Typical policies provided for comprehensive medical and hospital care in return for a fixed fee, which was divided between employer and employee. The insurance companies, called hospital asso-

[27]Goldberg and Greenberg, "The Effect of Physician-Controlled Health Insurance," p. 49.

[28]Goldberg and Greenberg, "The Emergence of Physician-Sponsored Health Insurance," p. 289.

[29]Ibid.

ciations, were originally begun by physicians but were later managed by lay personnel. Some associations owned their own hospitals, and others used the facilities of community hospitals. Since many of the associations were profit-making institutions, they had excellent incentives to control medical costs.

Moreover, there is ample evidence that the hospital associations aggressively monitored medical services in order to keep costs down. Physicians' fees were scrutinized closely. Doctors were often warned about unnecessary surgery and were frequently asked to justify their procedures. Length of stay in the hospital was another concern. Physicians were often asked to explain or justify hospital stays that were out of line with the average stays for particular procedures.

The following letter, sent by the Industrial Hospital Association to Oregon physicians in 1935, typifies the tough attitude of the insurers of the period:

> We solicit your cooperation in adhering to the following regulations:
>
> 1. All cases requiring major surgery, except in actual emergency, must be reported to the Association for authority before the operation is performed.
> 2. It will be the policy of the Association to require consultation before authorizing major surgery.
> 3. No operation for hernia will be authorized until the same has been approved by the State Industrial Accident Commission or the Association has had the opportunity to make satisfactory investigation.
> 4. Hospital ticket or treatment order must be obtained in advance of giving treatments, except in the cases of actual emergencies. No bills will be paid without tickets being attached.[30]

Two features of the hospital association's practices were especially irritating to physicians. First, the associations in effect limited the doctors' freedom of action. Physicians traditionally have not been accustomed to, and do not like, third parties interfering with their decisions about medical procedures. Second, the associations limited the ability of physicians to price discriminate. The associations were not inclined to pay higher fees simply because physicians decided that they could afford them. Nevertheless, a great many doctors cooperated with the hospital associations, primarily for financial reasons. The associations guaranteed payment for medical services rendered, payment that might otherwise not have been received. This guarantee was especially important during the years of the Great Depression.

30Reprinted in Goldberg and Greenberg, "The Emergence of Physician-Sponsored Health Insurance," p. 294.

Enter the forces of organized medicine. The opposition of organized medicine to the for-profit hospital associations in Oregon had two distinct stages. In the first, prior to 1941, the strategy for undermining the associations consisted of (1) policy statements warning physicians that "contract medicine" was unethical; (2) the formation of rival prepaid plans sponsored by county medical bureaus; and (3) the expulsion of "unethical" physicians from county medical societies. In the second stage, beginning in 1941, organized medicine created its own statewide insurance company, the Oregon Physicians' Service (OPS). OPS was the forerunner of the current Blue Shield system in Oregon.

Once OPS was established, organized medicine was in a position to abandon its concerted effort to keep physicians from dealing with the hospital associations. To make OPS attractive to patients, complete freedom of choice of physicians was allowed. Rates were kept low by keeping a tight lid on reimbursements to physicians. OPS was even given permission to advertise. To make the plan attractive to doctors, OPS operations were generally placed under the control of county medical societies, but there was no interference with the medical decisions of doctors. OPS did not, however, always pay what the physician billed.

OPS grew rapidly. By the middle of the first year of operation, 95 percent of the membership of the Oregon State Medical Society and 85 percent of all practicing physicians in Oregon belonged to OPS. An ever-increasing number of patients joined as well. By 1948 the three remaining for-profit hospital associations made approximately 24 percent of total health insurance disbursements — down from 51 percent of all disbursements at the end of 1940. Moreover, during this period the total level of health insurance disbursements increased 500 percent. As the number of patients with OPS coverage grew, the system became increasingly attractive to physicians, but physicians were not allowed to be members of OPS unless they were members in good standing of their local medical societies, and an implicit requirement for a good-standing rating was noncooperation with the hospital associations. This included joining a collective boycott against the competition.

Of particular importance was the policy of refusing to accept the tickets of patients who subscribed to the hospital association plans. A cooperating physician would take such a ticket and bill the hospital association directly, but a noncooperating physician would refuse the ticket and bill the patient. The patient could then seek reimbursement from the association, but if the association's reimbursement was less than the patient's charge, the association would find itself in disfavor with the patient.

In response to this challenge, the hospital associations began to liberalize their cost-curtailing policies. They began to allow patients the freedom to choose their physician and ceased interfering with the medical decisions of doctors. As a result, the insurance market in Oregon gradually evolved into the same type of medical insurance market that exists elsewhere. Goldberg and Greenberg summarize this evolution:

> Though their market shares decreased, the three for-profit associations were able to continue in the market by changing their methods of operation. The elimination of severe competitive pressures enabled the hospital associations to lead the "quiet life" under an OPS umbrella. In addition, in the early 1950s the commercial insurance companies entered the prepaid health insurance market in Oregon and by 1957 were able to secure more than half the total membership in all health plans. *We have found no evidence that these firms acted aggressively to control costs.*[31]

The Role of Blue Cross and Blue Shield

The health insurance market in the United States has two primary components. First is the commercial, competitive part of the market, consisting of over 300 firms. This component is relatively unconcentrated, and entry into it appears to be relatively easy. On the buyer's side of the market, over 85 percent of the individuals insured for hospital expenses are covered by group policies, usually purchased through employers. The market, therefore, appears to be dominated by relatively informed buyers, and, on the whole, is relatively competitive.[32]

The other component consists of Blue Cross and Blue Shield plans. These plans were originally created by providers of health services and are alleged to be controlled and operated in the interest of the providers. Blue Cross was created by hospitals to provide hospital insurance; Blue Shield was created by physicians to provide physicians'-services insurance.[33] State Blue Cross–Blue Shield enabling acts have typically required that such plans be subject to medical society approval or that a

31Ibid., p. 313. Emphasis added.

32H. E. Frech and Paul Ginsburg, "Competition Among Health Insurers," *Competition in the Health Care Sector*, p. 211.

33See Rayack, pp. 157–58 and pp. 46–54.

TABLE 5.1

Representation on Blue Cross and Blue Shield Governing Boards

Year	The public[1]	Medical people[2]	Hospital people[3]
	Representation on Blue Cross Governing Boards (in percentages)		
1959	32	17	51
1964	41	16	43
	Representation on Blue Shield Governing Boards (in percentages)		
1959	25	61	14
1964	31	63	6

SOURCE: *Medical Economics*, June 28, 1965, p. 75. Copyright © 1965 by Litton Industries, Inc. Published by Medical Economics Co., a Litton division, at Oradell, NJ 07649. Reprinted by permission. Data presented by the National Association of Blue Shield Plans and the Blue Cross Association.

[1]Farm, labor, and general representatives.

[2]Physicians and lay executives of sponsoring medical societies.

[3]Hospital trustees and administrators.

majority of the board of directors be physicians.[34] Local hospitals often advanced the initial capital for such plans,[35] and Blue Shield has been frequently publicized as "the doctor's plan — *for the people.*" (The emphasis is Blue Shield's.) Although the proportion of provider representation on the board of directors of such plans has declined in recent years, table 5.1 shows that physician and hospital dominance of the Blues continues to exist.

Whether Blue Cross and Blue Shield plans function exclusively in the interests of organized medicine has been questioned.[36] The fact that many individual physicians object to specific policies of these organizations is largely irrelevant. Any organization that pursues group goals will naturally, at some time or other, find itself in conflict with individual members. If the Blues do not serve the monopolistic

[34]Herman Somers and Anne Somers, *Doctors, Patients and Health Insurance* (Washington, D.C.: Brookings Institution, 1961).

[35]Louis Reed, *Blue Cross and Medical Service Plans* (Washington, D.C.: Federal Security Agency, U.S. Public Health Service, 1947), p. 13.

[36]See Odin Anderson, *Blue Cross Since 1929* (Cambridge, Mass.: Ballinger Publishing Co., 1975).

TABLE 5.2

Blue Cross and Blue Shield Market Share[1]

Year	Regular Medical Insurance	Hospital Expense Insurance	Year	Regular Medical Insurance	Hospital Expense Insurance
1940	0.066	0.488	1966	0.436	0.428
1945	0.276	0.589	1967	0.434	0.427
1950	0.512	0.489	1968	0.434	0.429
1955	0.517	0.466	1969	0.425	0.429
1960	0.504	0.437	1970	0.421	0.433
1961	0.483	0.431	1971	0.426	0.433
1962	0.478	0.432	1972	0.428	0.432
1963	0.463	0.428	1973	0.421	0.435
1964	0.449	0.427	1974	0.416	0.435
1965	0.441	0.427			

SOURCE: *Sourcebook of Health Insurance Data, 1975–1976.*

[1]Based on numbers of individuals insured.

goals of organized medicine, they certainly possess the potential to do so.[37]

Unlike the commercial side of the health insurance market, the Blue Cross–Blue Shield side is characterized by monopoly. In many states the Blues are organized under special enabling acts that restrict additional entry into this part of the market.[38] As table 5.2 shows, the share of the total insurance market held by the Blues has been remarkably stable in recent years. Moreover, within this part of the market there is a great deal of collusion. Frech and Ginsberg describe this market in the following way:

> The Blues collude almost perfectly. Blue Cross and Blue Shield plans agree upon geographical market areas with the assistance of their national associations. Further, with few exceptions, the local Blue Cross plan agrees not to sell physician service insurance, while the local Blue Shield plan agrees not to sell hospital insurance. This means that, from a national antitrust perspective, we can treat the entire Blue Cross/Blue Shield complex as one firm.[39]

The market power of the Blues varies immensely from state to state. Some states have almost no Blue Cross or Blue Shield insurance plans,

[37]See Sloan and Feldman, pp. 93 ff.

[38]Frech and Ginsburg, p. 211.

[39]Ibid., p. 212.

while in others the Blues have market shares that reach as high as 80 percent.[40] What accounts for the large market share of the Blues in those states where they flourish? The most basic explanation is regulation.

Insurance regulation is enacted at the state level, and in various ways most state insurance regulations confer competitive advantages on the Blues. For example, in most states taxes are assessed on insurance premiums, and the revenue is used to finance the regulatory apparatus. In a majority of states, however, the Blues pay lower taxes — on the order of 2 to 3 percent of premiums — or no taxes at all.[41] To gauge the effect of this advantage, consider the fact that net revenues (premiums minus benefit payments) on group policies are usually less than 10 percent of the total premiums. This is the income with which the insurers cover their costs. Note that a 2 to 3 percent premium tax differential is equal to about 20 to 30 percent of net revenues.[42]

The Blues are also often exempted from other taxes, such as real estate taxes. In some states commercial insurance policies sold to individuals are required to meet minimum benefit/premium rates, whereas Blue Cross-Blue Shield policies are not. Other states regulate the rates charged by the Blues, but in terms of overall premium rather than in terms of a benefit/premium rate. In most states required reserves are also lower or nonexistent for the Blues.[43]

Given these regulatory advantages, it is surprising that the blues have not captured the entire market for health insurance. Some economists have argued that one reason they have not is that the Blues use their advantages to pursue nonpecuniary goals, some of which are important to organized medicine.[44] The most dramatic instance of the use of market power to prevent commercial insurance from pursuing an activist claims review is the Oregon case, summarized in the previous section. It is not known whether the Blues have used their market power to achieve similar ends in recent years. What is known is that the Blues — as well as the commercial health insurance firms — are remarkably lax in reviewing claims, at least in comparison with the insurance market in other fields.

It is possible that the mere existence of the Blues poses a potential

[40]Ibid.

[41]David Robbins, "Comment" in *Competition in the Health Care Sector*, p. 263.

[42]Frech and Ginsburg, p. 214.

[43]Ibid.

[44]Ibid., pp. 216–19.

threat to the commercial insurance companies and that this threat is sufficient to discipline the latter's behavior. Take the case of Aetna. In the early 1970s Aetna Life and Casualty Company, with nearly twelve million policyholders, attempted to hold down medical costs by injecting itself into doctor-patient disputes. At that time Aetna had agreements with its usual and customary policyholders stating that where:

> *1.* Aetna disallowed a portion of the fee for exceeding prevailing limits;
>
> *2.* attempts to resolve the difference with the doctor failed;
>
> *3.* the patient refused to pay the balance himself; and
>
> *4.* the doctor sued the patient for the balance,

Aetna would pay to defend the suit.[45] Aetna also sent form letters to policyholders whose claims were not fully paid by Aetna notifying them that their doctors were charging more than the prevailing rates in their area.

What followed was a storm of protest from the medical community. In June 1972 the AMA convention adopted a resolution condemning the Aetna policy and calling for meetings between AMA and Aetna representatives "to satisfactorily resolve the problem."[46] Such meetings did occur. And, in a startling reversal of policy, in a meeting between representatives of Aetna and the AMA, Aetna affirmed the following:

> *1.* Aetna has discontinued a standard practice of sending letters to patients offering to pay legal expenses should legal action be brought against one of its insureds.... It never has been and is not now Aetna's policy to encourage or to aid its insureds to bring legal action against physicians.
>
> *2.* In the event a physician's charge exceeds in a significant amount Aetna's calculation of the upper limit of the range of prevailing fees for the procedure performed, Aetna will contact the physician prior to communicating its benefit determination to the claimant; however, contact will not necessarily be made when an

[45]Charlotte L. Rosenberg, "He Challenged Aetna's Hard-line Fee Policy — and Won," *Medical Economics*, 11 September 1972, p. 31.

[46]Ibid., p. 34.

individual physician's usual charge has been documented through past experience as routinely above the prevailing range as calculated by Aetna....

3. When, following discussion with the physician, Aetna is unable to accept the full amount of a charge as within the range of prevailing fees, it will ordinarily seek the advice of a peer review committee or other review mechanism of the appropriate medical society before finally determining its benefit payment....

4. In any instance involving a question of types of treatments, alternative types of services, or volume of services ordered or provided, it is the policy of Aetna to make inquiry of the physician first and, if necessary, to seek supplemental advice through peer review....[47]

As a result of this policy reversal, Aetna today apparently does little to reduce physician charges or to limit unnecessary procedures.[48]

The Economic Effects of AMA Policies Toward Medical Insurance

The policies of organized medicine toward health insurance have contributed to waste and inefficiency in the market for medical care, and, in the process, have been a major factor contributing to the rising costs of that care. These policies achieve their effects by producing distortions on both the demand and the supply side of the market.

Lack of Restraints on Suppliers' Costs The current attitude of insurance companies toward physician and hospital charges, as we have seen, is quite different from the conditions that existed when the hospital associations of Oregon competed in a free health insurance market. One recent study summarized current conditions:

> In few major industries is there such widespread use of non-negotiated, cost-based reimbursement. For more than 50 percent of the dollars spent for hospital care, the hospital need only justify that it actually incurred a legitimate health-care expense and the money will be paid. For most of the remaining bills, an insurance company is required to pay whatever the hospital feels is an appropriate charge for its service. The market is such that insurance companies

[47]Aetna Affidavit, Exhibit D. *State of Ohio* v. *Ohio Medical Indemnity*, Ind., Cir. No. 2-75-473 (S.D. Ohio, filed July 9, 1975). Reprinted in Goldberg and Greenberg, "The Effect of Physician-Controlled Health Insurance," pp. 64–65.

[48]Ibid., p. 65.

are forced to pay whatever the institutions selected by its policyholders [most likely selected by their physicians] charge for the services covered in the policy.[49]

Lack of Restraints on Physician Procedures Equally serious is the problem of a physician's discretion on the use of certain procedures. In the 1930s the hospital associations of Oregon didn't pay for an appendectomy just because a physician felt like performing one. The associations often demanded to know precisely what conditions justified the surgery. In today's insurance market things are quite different. Table 5.3 compares surgical rates of neighboring towns in Vermont that have comparable populations and insurance coverage. As the table shows, per capita surgery rates vary up to 200 percent overall and up to 300 percent for specific procedures.[50] No apparent explanation exists for these variations aside from the predilections of individual doctors and hospitals for certain types of procedures.

Ample evidence suggests that surgical rates vary dramatically in response to variations in the financial incentives faced by doctors. One study found large and significant differences in hospital and surgical utilization rates between Medicaid beneficiaries served by group-practice HMOs and control groups served by fee-for-service physicians.[51] No significant difference was found between the two groups of patients in terms of perceived health status, the number of chronic conditions, or the number of disability days per month. There was, however, a major difference in the financial incentives faced by doctors: Fee-for-service physicians have an incentive to overprovide services, whereas physicians working under HMOs have an incentive to underprovide services. Other studies have noted similar differences between federal employees and their families cared for by group-

49Stuart Altman and Sanford Weiner, "Regulation as a Second Best," in *Competition in the Health Care Sector*, p. 426, n. 1.

50For additional evidence on widespread variations in surgical rates see J. P. Bunker, "Surgical Manpower: A Comparison of Operations and Surgeons in the United States, England, and Wales," *New England Journal of Medicine* 282 (January 1970): 135–44; Paul Lembke, "Measuring the Quality of Medical Care Through Vital Statistics Based on Hospital Service Areas: A Comparative Study of Appendectomy Rates," *American Journal of Public Health* 42 (March 1952): 276–86; and John Wennberg, "Testimony and Statement," in *Getting Ready for National Health Insurance: Unnecessary Surgery*, hearings before the Subcommittee on Oversight and Investigations of the Committee on Interstate and Foreign Commerce, U.S. House of Representatives, 94th Congress, Serial No. 94–37, 15 July 1975.

51Clifton Gares, B. Cooper, and C. Hirschman, "Contrast in HMO and Fee-for-Service Performance," *Social Security Bulletin*, May 1976, pp. 3–14.

TABLE 5.3

Variation in Number of Surgical Procedures Performed per 10,000 Persons for the 13 Vermont Hospital Service Areas and Comparison Populations, Vermont, 1969[1]

Surgical Procedure	Lowest Two Areas		Entire State	Highest Two Areas	
All Surgery	360	490	550	610	690
Tonsillectomy	13	32	43	85	151
Appendectomy	10	15	18	27	32
Hemorrhoidectomy	2	4	6	9	10
Males					
Hernioplasty	29	38	41	47	48
Prostatectomy	11	13	20	28	38
Females					
Cholecystectomy	17	19	27	46	57
Hysterectomy	20	22	30	34	60
Mastectomy	12	14	18	28	33
Dilation and curettage	30	42	55	108	141
Varicose veins	6	7	12	24	28

SOURCE: J. Wennberg, "PSRO and the Relationships among Health Need, Elective Surgery and Health Status," *Perspectives on Health Policy* (Boston: Boston University Medical Center, 1975). Reprinted by permission.

[1]Rates adjusted to Vermont age composition.

practice HMOs and those cared for under fee-for-service arrangements.[52]

Lack of Restraints on Patient Demand One of the most serious problems in the health care market today is that consumers of medical services have poor financial incentives to exercise restraint in the consumption of those services. Table 5.4 shows why. Between 1950 and 1975, average cost per patient per day in a hospital increased about 1,000 percent. In real terms the increase was over 450 percent. The patients themselves have not borne these dramatic increases in the form of out-of-pocket medical expenses, however. In 1950 insurance plus government aid paid about half of the hospital bill. In 1975, however, third-party payers assumed about 90 percent of the bill. What this means to the consumer is indicated by the final entry in table 5.4. Despite the fact that a hospital in 1975 had a far greater amount of

[52]See, for example, George Monsma, "Marginal Revenue and the Demand for Physicians' Services," in Herbert Klarman, ed., *Empirical Studies in Health Economics* (Baltimore: Johns Hopkins University Press, 1970).

TABLE 5.4

Insurance and the Net Cost of Hospital Care
(Short-term, Non-Federal, General Hospitals)

	1950	1955	1960	1966	1970	1972	1974	1975
Percentage of costs paid by:								
Private insurance	29.3	44.7	52.5	51.4	45.6	45.4	45.4	43.6
Government	21.1	19.9	18.8	25.5	37.8	41.1	42.8	44.5
Direct consumer spending	49.6	35.2	28.7	23.1	16.6	13.5	11.8	11.9
Average cost per patient day	15.62	23.12	32.23	48.15	81.01	105.21	128.05	151.53
Net consumer cost per patient day	7.75	8.14	9.25	11.12	13.53	14.20	15.11	18.03
Average cost per patient day (1967 dollars)	21.66	28.83	36.34	49.54	69.66	83.97	86.70	94.00
Net consumer cost per patient day (1967 dollars)	10.75	10.15	10.43	11.44	11.63	11.34	10.23	11.18

SOURCE: Martin Feldstein and Amy Taylor, *The Rapid Rise of Hospital Costs* (Cambridge, Mass: Harvard Institute of Economic Research, Harvard University, 1977), tables 8 and 9. Reprinted by permission.

services and a much higher quality of care to offer patients than did a hospital in 1950, the out-of-pocket expense borne by patients for a day in the hospital in 1975 was, in real terms, only forty-three cents more than it was in 1950. Third-party payments for outpatient physician's services are not quite as extensive, amounting currently to about 60 percent of total charges.[53]

Even if we disregard Medicare, Medicaid, and other government programs, the picture does not change much. In 1950 private insurance paid about 37 percent of all private hospital bills. By 1975 private insurance was paying for 79 percent of privately-financed hospital care, which means that, in real terms, patients with private insurance policies were paying only four dollars more in out-of-pocket expense for a day in the hospital in 1975 than they were in 1950.[54]

One way or another, consumers wind up footing the total cost of hospital care. In addition to out-of-pocket expenses, they pay higher insurance premiums and higher taxes to cover the increasing hospital costs. The costs that affect patient behavior, however, are not *total* but *marginal* costs. In making the decision to consume ten dollars of additional hospital care, the average patient today will incur only one dollar of additional *personal* expense, and the average privately-insured patient will incur only two dollars of additional *personal* expense.

The coronary bypass operation provides a dramatic example of how third-party payments distort the incentives patients face. This operation costs $10,000 and up and has generated considerable controversy because some doctors believe its cost often far exceeds its value. The average patient, however, need not realize $10,000 worth of benefit in order to make the operation worthwhile to him; he need only be willing to pay an additional $1,000 out of pocket in order to hedge his bets.

The problem of distorted patient incentives under insurance, generally known as the problem of "moral hazard," has been extensively analyzed by economists since it was first formally addressed by Kenneth Arrow over sixteen years ago.[55] In general the most effective way of minimizing the problem is by raising the out-of-pocket costs borne by patients at the point at which they consume hospital services,

[53]Altman and Weiner, p. 426.

[54]Martin Feldstein, "The High Cost of Hospitals — and What to Do About It," *Public Interest* 48 (1977): 42.

[55]Kenneth Arrow, "Uncertainty and the Welfare Economics of Medical Care," *American Economic Review* 53 (December 1963): 941–73.

which can be accomplished by raising deductibles and coinsurance rates (the percentage of charges paid by the patient). In fact, however, the trend in health insurance has been in the opposite direction — toward lower deductibles and lower coinsurance rates.

Organized medicine has contributed to this trend in two ways. The first is through the insurance strategy of Blue Cross and Blue Shield: A number of investigators have pointed out that the Blues prefer more complete insurance coverage because wider coverage serves the interests of organized medicine by increasing the demand for medical services.[56] One recent study has furnished evidence that the Blues use their market power (thus sacrificing "profits") to induce the public to accept more complete insurance than consumers would otherwise prefer.[57]

A second way that organized medicine has contributed to more complete insurance coverage is through political support of federal tax policies that encourage such coverage. Consider a family of four with an income of only $8,000 per year. If the husband's employer raises his pay by $100, income and payroll taxes will claim about $30, leaving the employee with only $70 in take-home pay. On the other hand, if the employer uses the $100 to purchase additional health insurance, the worker gains the full $100 in the form of insurance premiums. In dollar amounts, the employee gets 50 percent more if his employer chooses more health insurance instead of higher wages.[58] The incentives to acquire additional health insurance are even greater for moderate- and high-income employees. Moreover, when individuals purchase more health insurance on their own, they can usually deduct about one-half of the premiums from their federal income tax.

These provisions of federal law are often referred to as tax subsidies, and by some estimates the tax subsidy for individual purchases of health insurance amounts to $6 billion a year.[59] The term "tax subsidy" is misleading, however, because it implies that an individual's income belongs to the government and that the government is subsidizing him if it does not take the income to which it is entitled. Without endorsing this view, we can nonetheless concur that federal tax policies distort the incentives faced by the public and thus exacerbate the problem of over-insurance in health care.

[56]Sloan and Feldman, pp. 94–98; and Frech and Ginsburg, pp. 212–13 and pp. 216–19.

[57]Frech and Ginsburg, pp. 216–19.

[58]Feldstein, p. 45.

[59]Ibid.

VI. THE EFFECTS OF PROFESSIONAL CONTROL: PROVIDERS VERSUS THE PUBLIC

Each of us is a producer and also a consumer. However, we are much more specialized and devote a much larger fraction of our attentions to our activity as a producer than as a consumer. We consume literally thousands if not millions of items. The result is that people in the same trade, like barbers or physicians, all have an intense interest in the specific problems of this trade and are willing to devote considerable energy to doing something about them. . . . The groups that have a special interest . . . are concentrated groups to whom the issue makes a great deal of difference. The public interest is widely dispersed. In consequence, in the absence of any general arrangements to offset the pressure of special interests, producer groups will invariably have a much stronger influence on legislative action and the powers that be than the widely spread consumer interest. Indeed from this point of view, the puzzle is not that we have so many silly licensure laws, but why we don't have far more. The puzzle is how we ever succeeded in getting the relative freedom from government controls over the productive activities of individuals that we have had and still have in this country, and that other countries have had as well.

Milton Friedman
Capitalism and Freedom

In the previous chapters we have seen that organized medicine has used the coercive powers of government to promote the financial self-interest of physicians in many ways. By influencing the enactment of stiff licensing laws and by controlling the nation's medical schools, the AMA has succeeded in erecting formidable entry barriers to prospective physicians. Licensing laws have also been instrumental in preventing nurses and other paraprofessional personnel from performing tasks they are perfectly capable of performing in a safe and satisfactory manner, but which would enlarge the supply of physicians' services and thus lessen the financial return to the practice of medicine. By maintaining control of the accreditation of internship and residency programs, organized medicine has played an unclear, but probably substantial, role in the demise of the proprietary hospital and in the limiting of competition among public and voluntary hospitals. Through the use of both state regulatory powers and government-derived monopoly powers, organized medicine has curtailed the inclination of commercial health insurance companies to review claims aggressively and control medical costs.

A primary objective of organized medicine has been to maximize the income of physicians by maintaining an effective cartel among medical care providers. The cartel functions not only to maintain a monopolistic pricing structure for medical services, but also to price discriminate among patients with differing demands for those services. Organized medicine has attempted to pursue these objectives by disciplining those providers who compete for patients by cutting prices, by advertising, or by using any other technique that threatens to undermine the cartel. It has used its powers of license suspension and/or revocation and its control over access to hospitals to discipline individual physicians. Its control over hospital accreditation for physicians' training programs, as well as its influence in government regulatory agencies, serves as a threat to hospital managers who otherwise might be tempted to compete aggressively for patients. In some instances it has used the regulatory powers of the state to outlaw prepaid insurance schemes and in other instances to promote a health insurance market in which errant insurance companies are threatened with extinction if they challenge AMA-sanctioned policies.

How has the market for medical care been affected, overall, by the power of organized medicine? In this chapter we will briefly consider the impact of AMA policies on physicians' incomes and health care costs.

Physicians' Incomes

Given the apparent power of organized medicine to control supplier behavior in the medical marketplace, it might seem that the practice of medicine would be extremely profitable. It is true that physicians have high incomes — about five times as high as the average wage paid in manufacturing — but when their incomes are matched against the investment required for their training, the profitability of medical practice is rather modest. How can this be? Consider the analogies provided by two other markets in which a long history of government intervention intended to raise the producer's profit has had little positive effect: airlines and oil.

Since 1938 the Civil Aeronautics Board (CAB) appears to have had one overriding objective: to secure a "reasonable" or "fair" rate of return for the commercial airline companies. This objective was pursued in two principal ways: by prohibiting new entry into the market and by keeping airline fares high above the competitive level. In its first forty years of operation, the CAB did not allow a single new carrier into the interstate market.[1] One economic study estimated that between 1969 and 1974 first class and coach fares would have been from 22 to 52 percent lower without CAB price regulation.[2]

Despite these efforts the rate of return on invested capital in the airline industry in the years prior to the recent deregulation efforts was, on the average, less than the average rate of return for all manufacturing industries.[3] The major reason that the airlines were not more profitable is that they engaged in costly quality competition. Unable to compete with each other on the basis of price, the airlines competed by scheduling more flights between cities and by providing costly amenities to attract customers. Because the airlines were unable to compete to bring price down to the level of average production costs, they simply reversed the process: They competed to bring average cost up to the level of price. CAB regulations were costly to consumers — about $2 billion per year by one estimate — but the airlines apparently realized very little long-run benefit.[4]

A similar phenomenon occurred in the oil industry. Prior to the Arab oil embargo of 1973, the oil industry had managed over the years to secure a series of favorable regulations designed to raise oil company profits. The depletion allowance was the most notorious of these: Producers were able to take large tax deductions that bore no relationship to any production costs they incurred. Less well known, but probably more lucrative, was the IRS treatment of intangible drilling costs — the deductions allowed here were way out of line with tax policy in other industries. In addition, the government instituted an import quota system in 1959 that limited the amount of foreign oil brought into the United States. Import licenses, required for all foreign oil, were

[1]John Goodman and Edwin Dolan, *Economics of Public Policy: The Micro View* (St. Paul: West Publishing Co., 1979), p. 148.

[2]Comptroller General of the United States.

[3]George W. Douglas, "Regulation of the U.S. Airline Industry: An Interpretation," in James Miller III, ed., *Perspectives on Federal Transportation Policy* (Washington, D.C.: American Enterprise Institute for Public Policy Research, 1975), pp. 71–83.

[4]Comptroller General of the United States.

simply given to the oil companies under a formula that ensured that most of the import rights went to the largest oil companies. The value of this subsidy has been estimated at $1 million per day. Congress also put its stamp of approval on the Oil Compact, a euphemism for a domestic oil cartel. Under this arrangement, regulatory commissions in such states as Texas, Louisiana, and Oklahoma were allowed to formulate coordinated policies designed to keep oil production down and oil prices up, all for the benefit of producers in the industry.[5]

The government, then, granted a great many favors to the oil producers, but it did not control the many ways that companies could spend money to compete with each other. Like airline regulation, government regulation of oil was costly to consumers, but it did little to improve the long-run profits of the producers. The ten-year (1963–72) average return on net wealth in petroleum production and refining was only 11.7 percent, while the average for all U.S. manufacturing companies for the same period was 12.2 percent.[6] Apparently political favoritism produced only temporary gains that quickly evaporated as many firms competed to enjoy them.

Like regulation in the airline and oil industries, regulation of the medical marketplace has been more costly to consumers than it has been profitable for physicians. Although physicians fees have been high, individual practitioners have responded by working longer hours, by taking more years of postgraduate training, and by incurring larger outlays for office equipment and services designed to attract patients.

One way of assessing the profitability of medicine is to treat the investment in medical training like any other investment and ask what rate of return the prospective medical student can expect to receive.[7] Health economist Keith Leffler has recently done this, and his results are shown in the second column of table 6.1. Leffler's estimates show what rate of return a college graduate, age twenty-two, can expect to earn if he embarks on a career as a general practitioner in each of the indicated years. In calculating the estimates, Leffler made adjustments for number of hours worked, length of training period, anticipated

[5]Goodman and Dolan, pp. 120–21.

[6]Shyam Sunder, *Oil Industry Profits* (Washington, D.C.: American Enterprise Institute for Public Policy Research, 1977), p. 67.

[7]An *internal rate of return* on an investment is that interest rate which makes the present worth of future income equal to the investment's cost.

TABLE 6.1

Internal Rate of Return and Profitability at 10 Percent Discount Rate of Five Years of Medical Training, Selected Years 1947–1973

Year	Internal Rate of Return[1] (Percent)	Profitability[2]	Year	Internal Rate of Return[1] (Percent)	Profitability[2]
1947	7	11,464	1967	14	32,610
1951	10½	2,622	1969	14	29,389
1955	10	2,003	1970	15	37,904
1959	10½	4,542	1971	15½	38,369
1961	11	7,015	1972	14	26,040
1963	11½	9,739	1973	15	30,740
1965	12	15,366			

SOURCE: Keith Leffler, *Explanations in Search of Facts: A Critique of "A Study of Physicians' Fees,"* (Coral Gables, Florida: Law and Economics Center, University of Miami School of Law, 1978), table 4, p. 12. Reprinted by permission.

[1]Estimated to closest ½ percent.

[2]Real (1976=100) dollars.

mortality, progressive income taxation, probability of being drafted, and tuition and scholarships at medical schools.[8]

As table 6.1 shows, the rate of return to medical training was 7 percent in 1947, 10 to 12 percent between 1951 and 1965, and 14 to 15.5 percent thereafter. To evaluate these numbers it is necessary to compare them to the rate of return paid on comparable investments, such as undergraduate education. Estimates of the rate of return from undergraduate education range from 8 to 13 percent.[9] Prior to the introduction of Medicaid and Medicare in 1965, then, rates of return on medical education appear to have been quite reasonable.

The third column in table 6.1 presents another way of looking at the profitability of medical training. This column gives estimates of the value of admission to medical school at a 10 percent rate of discount. As the numbers show, the profitability of medical school training was quite modest prior to the introduction of Medicaid and Medicare, ranging from $2,003 to $9,739 between 1951 and 1965.

[8]See Keith Leffler, *Explanations in Search of Facts: A Critique of "A Study of Physicians' Fees,"* (Coral Gables, Florida: Law and Economics Center, University of Miami School of Law, 1978), pp. 11–12.

[9]Ibid., p. 13.

The effects of Medicaid and Medicare on physicians' incomes have apparently been substantial. These effects are operating on the demand side of the market and not on the supply side, however, and thus they are largely independent of the restrictive policies of the AMA. In addition, it is possible that Leffler's estimates of the value of admission to medical school in the early 1970s are too high. They do not, for example, take into account the rapid increase in the number of foreign medical school graduates entering the United States during these years — probably in response to the high physicians' incomes generated by the Medicare and Medicaid programs. They do not take account, either, of the growth of substitute medical services, such as biofeedback therapy, competing at the periphery of the medical marketplace. And they do not take account of the recent expansion in medical school capacity, which has increased the annual output of physicians by 60 percent since 1965.[10] Each of these factors has led to an increase in the supply of physicians' services and thus can be expected to decrease the incomes of physicians. Since 1970 the incomes of general practitioners have not kept pace with inflation. Between 1970 and 1975, for example, there was a decline of 8 percent in real earnings for general practitioners.[11]

Medical Costs

What has been the overall effect on the costs of medical care of professional control over the medical marketplace? Virtually all health economists agree that restrictive AMA policies have substantially increased health care costs. Estimating precisely how much the activities of organized medicine have increased our health care bill is a near-to-impossible task — and no one has tried it. Nevertheless, insight into the magnitude of the effect can be gained by looking at some studies of specific restrictive practices.

Take the ban on advertising, for example. Although no one has studied the direct effect of this ban on physician and hospital fees, studies have been done in related fields. John Cady recently compared the experience of states that allow price advertising for prescription drugs with states that prohibit such advertising. He found little difference between these two groups of states in the range and quality of services offered by pharmacists, but there was a significant difference in prices. In 1976 consumers in states that prohibited advertising paid

[10]Ibid., p. 14.

[11]Ibid.

$380 million more for prescription drugs.[12] Similar studies, with comparable results, have been done on the market for eyeglasses.[13]

Studies have also been done on the effects of Blue Cross–Blue Shield domination of the market for health insurance. One study found that, on the average, the Blues' current market share causes hospital costs per patient per day to be about 10 percent higher than they otherwise would be. The distortion is much greater in those states where the Blues' share of the market reaches up to 80 percent. The study estimates that if the Blues achieved total dominance of the market, per diem charges would rise by more than 22 percent.[14] Of course, no one really knows what the effect would be of reverting to truly free market competition of the type that flourished in Oregon in the 1930s.

Numerous studies have also been made of the effects of so-called over-insurance, that is, excessive health insurance coverage induced by, among other things, federal income tax policy and Blue Cross–Blue Shield policies. Although there is some disagreement on how large these effects are, virtually all health economists believe that expanded health insurance bears some responsibility for increasing hospital costs.[15] A recent study by Martin Feldstein indicates the possible magnitude of this increase. Feldstein estimates that if third party coverage of hospital costs rises by just four percentage points — from 88 percent of charges to 92 percent — the per diem price of hospital care will rise by 37 percent.[16]

Studies of prepaid group plans, long opposed by organized medicine as unethical but nevertheless flourishing because of a number of important legal changes, also indicate that past AMA policies have been costly for consumers. Studies of HMOs, for example, show that their members have total medical costs that are from 10 to 40 percent

[12]John Cady, *Restricted Advertising and Competition: The Case of Retail Drugs* (Washington, D.C.: American Enterprise Institute for Public Policy Research, 1976), p. 20. See also John Cady, *Drugs on the Market: The Impact of Public Policy on the Retail Market for Prescription Drugs* (Lexington, Mass.: D.C. Heath and Co., 1975), p. 95.

[13]See Lee Benham, "The Effect of Advertising on the Price of Eyeglasses," *Journal of Law and Economics* 15 (October 1972): 338–39.

[14]H. E. Frech and Paul Ginsburg, "Competition Among Health Insurers," in Warren Greenberg, ed., *Competition in the Health Care Sector: Past, Present, and Future* (Germantown, Md.: Aspen Systems Corporation, 1978), p. 181.

[15]Stuart H. Altman and Sanford L. Weiner, "Regulation as a Second Best," in Greenberg, p. 343 ff. See also Martin Feldstein and Amy Taylor, *The Rapid Rise of Hospital Costs* (Cambridge, Mass.: Harvard Institute of Economic Research, 1977).

[16]Martin Feldstein, "Quality Change and the Demand for Hospital Care," *Econometrica* 45 (October 1977): 1699.

lower than the annual health costs for comparable groups covered by conventional insurance.[17] The reduction of health costs that accompanies membership in such plans may be a mixed blessing, however. HMOs have lower surgical rates, but it is not clear that all of the reduction is the result of the elimination of unnecessary surgery.[18] Nonetheless, the AMA's past policies have clearly deprived consumers of a less costly option.

The policies of organized medicine have also resulted in other costs that are hard to measure in money terms. In chapter 5 we noted that the current system of medical insurance, largely the product of AMA policies, has encouraged many small hospitals to offer a wide range of surgical services, despite the fact that certain services may be performed infrequently and result in higher mortality rates when they are. One recent study shows that the mortality rates are quite high at small hospitals that perform certain kinds of surgery infrequently.[19] Consumers rarely know these facts, however, because hospital mortality rates are not made public. Even though the public disclosure of this information would improve the efficiency of the health care market and save a great many lives as well, organized medicine ardently resists.[20]

Is Medical Licensing Necessary?

We have presented in this and in preceding chapters a number of examples of how professional control of the market for medical care imposes higher costs on consumers. Is it possible, however, that government intervention has also produced benefits for consumers? That is, has government intervention in the medical marketplace resulted in any improvements over what would have occurred in a free market?

The position of the AMA and a number of health economists is that consumers are too ignorant to make adequately informed choices about health care.[21] They argue that if the free market were allowed to

17Harold S. Luft, "How Do Health Maintenance Organizations Achieve Their Savings?" *New England Journal of Medicine* 298 (June 1978): 1337.

18HMOs are considered more fully in chapter 7.

19Harold S. Luft, John P. Bunker, and Alain C. Enthoven, "Should Operations be Regionalized?" *New England Journal of Medicine* 301 (December 1979): 1364–69.

20See Clark Havighurst, "Regulation of Health Facilities and Services by Certificate of Need," *Virginia Law Review* 59 (October 1973): 1163, n. 76. See, however, Clark Havighurst and Laurence R. Tancredi, "Medical Adversity Insurance: A No-Fault Approach to Medical Malpractice and Quality Assurance," *Milbank Memorial Fund Quarterly* 51 (1973): 131.

21See, for example, Uwe Reinhart, "Comment," in Greenberg, pp. 128–29.

allocate health care resources, consumers would often fall victim to quacks and charlatans. After all, so the argument goes, if consumers are ignorant about matters of quality, they will be unable to distinguish between good and bad doctors. Medical licensure and other forms of professional control, then, help ensure that consumers make the choices they would have made were they well-informed.

There are several problems with this argument. First, it is not clear that consumers, on the average, are any less well-informed about medical care than they are about numerous other products, for which the market seems to work quite well. Mark V. Pauly has recently observed, "I know even less about the works of a movie camera than I know about my own organs; yet I feel fairly confident in purchasing a camera for a given price as long as I know that there are at least a few experts in the market who are keeping the sellers reasonably honest."[22] Pauly has also persuasively argued that there is little reason to believe that a free market for most medical services cannot operate as successfully as a free market for most other goods and services.[23]

Second, even if there were a justification for government action on the question of quality, the licensing of physicians and hospitals is still completely unwarranted. As Milton Friedman pointed out almost two decades ago, if government must do something, it could simply provide consumers with the information it thinks they should have.[24] Rather than establish by law who may or may not practice medicine, government might *certify* the skills and abilities of medical providers. A common example of certification is the warning label on cigarette packages. Consumers are given the surgeon general's opinion, but they may also seek other opinions and ultimately make their own decisions.

Third, licensing as such has little effect on the amount of fraud in the medical marketplace. In fact, given the alleged "conspiracy of silence" and the plethora of sanctions that may be imposed on physicians who testify in medical malpractice suits, medical fraud may be more prevalent today than it would have been in the absence of medical licensure. The almost daily succession of Medicaid and Medicare scandals suggests that medical fraud may be widespread. There are

[22]Mark V. Pauly, "The Behavior of Nonprofit Hospital Monopolies: Alternative Models of the Hospital," in Clark Havighurst, ed., *Regulating Health Facilities Construction* (Washington, D.C.: American Enterprise Institute, 1974), pp. 145–46.

[23]See Mark V. Pauly, "Is Medical Care Different?" in Greenberg, pp. 11–35.

[24]Milton Friedman, *Capitalism and Freedom* (Chicago: University of Chicago Press, 1962), chapter 9.

also effective ways to expose it. Pennsylvania, for example, employs a number of "medical detectives" who pose as patients and attempt to uncover fraudulent practices.[25]

Finally, as we noted in chapter 2, no one has succeeded in providing convincing evidence that medical licensure has in fact improved the average *quality* of patient care. There is evidence that medical licensure has increased the *price* of medical care — a quite different effect from the stated objectives of the AMA and the state legislatures.

[25] "Medical Sleuths Help Pennsylvania to Deal with Incompetent Doctors," *Wall Street Journal*, 1 May 1979, p. 1.

VII. ENFORCED COMPETITION: HMOs

The concept of free *competition* enforced *by law is a grotesque contradiction in terms.*

Ayn Rand
Capitalism: The Unknown Ideal

As the United States entered the decade of the seventies, policy makers became increasingly concerned over the nation's health care system. Not only were medical expenditures rising faster than the national income, but largely because of the Medicare and Medicaid programs, the government's medical expenditures were rising much faster than medical expenditures generally. In 1960, for example, the share of hospital expenses financed by government was actually lower than it had been a decade earlier. Between 1960 and 1970, however, the share of the nation's total hospital bill borne by the government more than doubled — rising from 18.8% of all hospital expenses to 37.8% of all hospital expenses.[1]

Faced with the alternatives of pushing for more regulation or more competition, the Nixon administration favored the latter course. It pursued this objective, however, in a somewhat strange way. The federal government might have promoted competition in health care services by passing legislation that nullifed the many laws and restrictions imposed on the market by state governments. That is, the federal government might have used its powers to remove the many legal obstacles that keep a genuine free market from working. What it in fact did was something very different: It created exemptions, privileges, and even subsidies for a special kind of health care delivery organization that it hoped would successfully compete with the more traditional forms of health care delivery. The organizations so favored were called federally qualified health maintenance organizations.

How HMOs Are Structured

The term "health maintenance organization" (HMO) was either coined or popularized by Dr. Paul M. Ellwood, Jr., the man generally

[1]See table 5.4.

credited with being the architect of the Nixon administration's program.[2] Although federal legislation provides a definition of an HMO, this definition is so restrictive as to exclude many organizations commonly thought to be HMOs. For the purposes of the present discussion, HMOs will be generally defined as organizations that assume a contractual obligation to provide or assure the delivery of health services to a voluntarily enrolled population paying a fixed premium.

HMOs, then, are essentially prepaid medical insurance plans. They are often classified in one of two ways, based on how physicians are paid.[3] "Closed-panel" HMOs reimburse physicians on a salaried or capitation basis and frequently operate as a group practice. "Medical care foundations," or "open-panel" HMOs, on the other hand, reimburse participating physicians on a fee-for-service basis, although such fees are limited by the total amount of prepayments collected from subscribers.[4]

Because they are prepaid plans, HMOs have different incentive structures than conventional insurance plans. Under conventional insurance plans, both the patient and the provider face incentives that tend to result in the overconsumption of medical care. The patient has an incentive to overconsume because he does not bear the full cost of the services he receives at the point of consumption. This incentive is reinforced by the fact that insurance companies do not risk-discriminate, i.e., the patient's premium does not rise because of his past consumption. Providers have no incentive to encourage patients to consume less because as the patients' consumption rises, so do provider incomes. In addition, physicians can increase their protection against malpractice suits by doing all that is "medically possible." Even when insurers are inclined to police insurance claims vigorously, they often find it costly to do so.

[2]See Clark C. Havighurst, "Health Maintenance Organizations and the Market for Health Services," *Health Care,* Library of Law and Contemporary Problems (Dobbs Ferry, N.Y.: Oceana, 1972), p. 719, n. 10.

[3]See Richard C. Augur and Victor P. Goldberg, "Prepaid Health Plans and Moral Hazard," *Public Policy* 22 (1974), pp. 353–63.

[4]Clearly, medical care foundations (MCFs) are more consistent with traditional fee-for-service medicine. In fact, MCFs have been sponsored by county medical societies and are open to all physician members of the society who agree to accept certain controls over their practice (maximum fees, peer reviews, etc.). Because of their sponsorship by organized medicine, some writers do not consider MCFs as legitimate HMOs. See Havighurst, "Health Maintenance Organizations and the Market for Health Services," p. 719 and p. 767.

In an HMO plan, consumers have an even greater incentive to overconsume because there is no deductible or coinsurance feature of the plan. But since HMOs furnish both insurance and medical care, the HMO itself has very different incentives than the fee-for-service providers. Once the premiums are paid, additional services do nothing more than increase costs, and therefore HMOs have an incentive to underprovide medical services. As Clark Havighurst has pointed out, in an extreme case an HMO has "a temptation to let a patient die of cardiac arrest rather than place him in the intensive care unit at a cost of $300 per day."[5]

This does not mean that HMOs intentionally allow their patients to die of cardiac arrests. For one thing, HMO physicians are subject to the same malpractice laws that apply to other physicians. For another, HMOs must compete for patients in the marketplace and the quality of the care administered is an obvious concern of potential customers.

What the incentive structure faced by HMOs does mean, however, is that HMO physicians and their patients face a potential conflict that does not exist, at least to the same extent, in the more traditional setting. In the HMO, patients may desire more care than physicians are willing to provide.[6] Most HMOs have a complaints procedure whereby patients may express grievances when conflicts do arise, however. In addition, the patients are always free to go outside the plan and purchase additional services if they desire.

How HMOs Work

How do HMOs actually work? Table 7.1 summarizes the evidence from five studies that compared the medical costs of enrollees in HMOs with comparable groups of people covered by conventional health insurance. Each of the studies included a California Kaiser-Permanente (HMO) plan, and these plans are therefore an excellent reference point in examining the results of the studies.

As table 7.1 shows, the basic premium charged by the Kaiser plans is sometimes higher than the premium charged by conventional insurance plans, which is understandable because under conventional

[5]Ibid., p. 723.

[6]For descriptions of the interaction between HMO physicians and "demanding" patients, see David Mechanic, *The Growth of Bureaucratic Medicine: An Inquiry into the Dynamics of Patient Behavior and the Organization of Medical Care* (New York: Wiley, 1976); and Eliott Freidson, "Prepaid Group Practice and the New 'Demanding Patient,'" *Health and Society*, Fall 1973, pp. 473–88.

insurance, people expect to bear out-of-pocket costs through deductibles and coinsurance payments. The table shows that Kaiser enrollees also bear some out-of-pocket costs, either because they purchased services not offered by Kaiser or because they wanted more service than Kaiser was willing to provide. Nonetheless, in each of the five studies, total medical care costs were lower for enrollees in the Kaiser HMO than in any of the other plans. Blue Cross–Blue Shield enrollees spent about 50% more (the range is from 16% to 88%) than Kaiser enrollees. People in indemnity insurance plans average about 21% (from 5% to 48%) more than Kaiser enrollees.

All of the available evidence, then, indicates that HMOs have the potential to reduce medical costs substantially, relative to conventional insurance. How do HMOs achieve these lower costs? There is no evidence, either theoretical or empirical, that HMOs provide services more efficiently than fee-for-service providers.[7] Both types of providers have the same inventive to do whatever they do at minimum cost. One recent study, for example, compared average length of hospitalization for certain procedures and found no difference between HMO patients and other patients.[8]

If there is no substantial difference in the efficiency of HMO and non-HMO providers, then the difference in costs must arise from a difference in the quantity or type of services delivered. Until recently it was widely believed that HMOs achieved their lower costs by eliminating unnecessary surgery. Conventional, fee-for-service physicians, it was alleged, often performed unneeded elective surgery. The frequent implication was that fraud, or near fraud, was involved. HMO physicians, on the other hand, had no financial incentive to perform such operations.[9]

These beliefs have been dispelled by a study by Professor Harold Luft of Stanford University. What Luft has shown is that HMOs have less hospitalization for every procedure. In particular, he showed that (1) HMOs reduce hospital admissions just as much for nonsurgical

[7]Harold S. Luft, "How do Health-Maintenance Organizations Achieve Their Savings?: Rhetoric and Evidence," *New England Journal of Medicine* 298 (15 June 1978): 1337.

[8]Ibid., p. 1339.

[9]See Larry Frederick, "How Much Unnecessary Surgery?: A Hard Look at the Evidence," *Medical World News* 17, no. 10 (1976), pp. 50–66; and United States House of Representatives, Subcommittee on Oversight and Investigations of the Committee on Interstate and Foreign Commerce, *Cost and Quality of Health Care: Unnecessary Surgery* (Washington, D.C.: U.S. Government Printing Office, 1976).

TABLE 7.1

Yearly Medical Care Expenditures per Person According to Type of Health Insurance Plan*

Plan	Premium	Direct Out-of-Pocket Costs	Total	Ratio of Total Cost to Lowest Total Cost in Study
Blue-collar union members, 1958†:				
Blue Cross–Blue Shield, NJ	$38	$51	$89	1.25
Major Medical-Indemnity	35–38	44	79–82	1.11–1.15
Kaiser†	39	32	71	1.00
Auto workers, Oakland, CA, 1959:				
Blue Cross–Blue Shield	$58	$63	$121	1.27
Kaiser†	57	38	95	1.00
CA state employees, 1962–63:				
Indemnity	$57	$47	$104	1.12
Blue Cross–Blue Shield	71	50	121	1.30
Kaiser†	71	22	93	1.00
Ross–Loos†	68	31	99	1.06
Individual practice associations‡	77	41	118	1.27
Enrollees in 6 Southern CA plans, 1967–68:				
Large commercial	$104	$79	$183	1.48
Small commercial	91	69	160	1.29
Blue Cross	127	108	235	1.90
Blue Shield	157	74	231	1.86
Kaiser†	111	13	124	1.00
Ross–Loos†	92	50	142	1.15
CA state employees, 1970/71:				
Indemnity plans	$102	$82	$184	1.05
Blue Cross–Blue Shield	160	89	249	1.42
Kaiser†	137	38	175	1.00
Ross–Loos/Family Health Plan†	140	63	203	1.16
Individual practice associations	128	89	217	1.24

SOURCE: Harold S. Luft, "How Do Health-Maintenance Organizations Achieve Their Savings?: Rhetoric and Evidence," *New England Journal of Medicine* 298, no. 24 (15 June 1978), p. 1337, table 1. Reprinted by permission.

*Methods vary from study to study, but are consistent across plans within each study.

†Prepaid group Practice ‡Medical care foundations

categories as for surgical categories, and (2) HMOs reduce surgical rates just as much for nonelective procedures as they do for elective procedures.[10]

Some of Luft's results are presented in table 7.2. The first eight columns of the table compare surgical rates in HMOs with the rates for conventional insurance enrollees for eight types of surgery often considered to be discretionary. The ninth column compares the surgical rates between the two groups for all surgical procedures. The only obvious exception to Luft's general conclusion is the differential between the ratio for tonsillectomies and for other forms of surgery. Luft reasons that the long standing controversy over tonsillectomies may have induced HMOs to subject these operations to particularly careful review.[11] The remaining seven types of discretionary operations, however, are split about evenly between those above and those below the overall ratios of HMO surgery to conventional surgery.

The inescapable conclusion is that HMOs clearly reduce medical costs by reducing all types of hospital procedures. What is not known is whether or not HMO patients are better or worse off than patients with conventional insurance. It may well be that such comparisons are meaningless. Perhaps the consumption of medical care is similar to the consumption of other goods and services — some people prefer to consume more and pay more, and others prefer to spend money elsewhere.[12]

What is important about HMOs is that, where they are allowed to do so, they can successfully compete in the marketplace. They can offer a lower-cost option to those patients who are willing to take fewer services in return. Clearly many people prefer this option. The most recent figures show that there are more than 200 HMOs operating in the United States, with a total membership of about 7.5 million people.[13]

[10]Luft, pp. 1340–41.

[11]Ibid., p. 1341.

[12]A possible exception to the rule that HMO patients are not obviously worse off is the recent experience with Medicaid (Medi-Cal) patients in California. In contrast to other states, California has encouraged Medicaid recipients to join HMOs called Prepaid Health Plans (PHPs). For a description of patient abuse under these plans, see Andreas G. Schneider and Joanne B. Stern, "Health Maintenance Organizations and the Poor: Problems and Prospects," *Northwestern University Law Review* 70 (1975): 130 f.

[13]"U.S. Increases Money Available to Health Maintenance Systems," *New York Times*, 13 April 1980.

TABLE 7.2

Comparison of Rates for Selected Procedures and Diagnoses in HMOs and Comparison Plans

Comparison	"Tonsil-lectomy"	"Hyster-ectomy"	"Hernia"	"Cholecys-tectomy"	"Cataract"	"Hemor-rhoid-ectomy"	"Prosta-tectomy"	"Varicose Veins"	All Surgical Procedures	All Admissions
	RATIO OF ADMISSION IN HMOS TO THOSE IN COMPARISON PLANS									
Health Insurance Plan/Blue Cross–Blue Shield	0.56	1.10	1.16	1.09	—	0.53	1.06	0.93	0.83	0.79
Health Insurance Plan/GHI* –males	—	—	0.69	0.92	—	0.11	2.08	—	0.95	0.93
Health Insurance Plan/GHI* –females	0.46	0.65	1.30	0.74	—	0.71	—	0.41	0.76	0.76
Health Insurance Plan/ union plan	0.69	0.76	0.77	0.87	—	0.95	—	0.88	—	0.98
Kaiser/Blue Cross–Blue Shield +indemnity	0.35	—	—	—	—	—	—	—	—	1.08
Federal employees–PGP†/ Blue Cross	0.35	0.52	0.71	—	—	—	—	—	0.45	—

(Cont. on p. 112)

TABLE 7.2 (CONTINUED)

Comparison	"Tonsil-lectomy"	"Hyster-ectomy"	"Hernia"	"Cholecys-tectomy"	"Cataract"	"Hemor-rhoid-ectomy"	"Prosta-tectomy"	"Varicose Veins"	All Surgical Procedures	All Admissions
	RATIO OF ADMISSION IN HMOS TO THOSE IN COMPARISON PLANS									
Group Health Centre/ indemnity	0.32	—	—	—	—	—	—	—	—	0.80
Group Health Association/ Blue Cross	0.25	—	0.83	0.55	—	—	0.57	—	—	0.53
Medical Care Group/ control	1.35	0.73	1.30	1.14	0.49	—	—	—	1.14	0.92

SOURCE: Harold S. Luft, "How Do Health-Maintenance Organizations Achieve Their Savings?: Rhetoric and Evidence," *New England Journal of Medicine* 298, no. 24 (15 June 1978), p. 1341, table 3. Reprinted by permission.

*Group Health Insurance, N.Y.

†Prepaid Group practice

State Government Restrictions on HMOs

Despite the fact that HMOs have flourished in some parts of the country for years, as of August 1973 less than half the states had at least one HMO in operation.[14] A general survey of state regulations in 1972 found that nine states prohibited HMOs altogether, and a total of twenty states either prohibited HMOs or had restrictions so severe that conventional HMOs could not operate. Among these restrictions were acts that required medical society approval of the articles of incorporation, medical society sponsorship or control of the directors or trustees of the plan, or actual medical society control of the plan itself.[15]

State laws proscribing the "corporate practice of medicine" represent another potential barrier because HMOs are corporations. In some states nonprofit HMOs are allowed to operate, while for-profit HMOs are prohibited. In addition, some state insurance regulations require HMOs to maintain large financial reserves and low insurance rates and to limit asset holdings. These laws, designed primarily for conventional health insurance programs, unfairly disadvantage HMOs because HMOs are providing benefits in-kind rather than in cash. Moreover, as we have seen, HMO premiums are often higher than conventional insurance premiums, even though HMOs seem to succeed in reducing overall medical costs for their enrollees.[16]

Another type of restriction on HMOs is represented by certificate-of-need laws. These laws, examined more thoroughly in chapter 8, often require HMOs to seek the approval of health planning agencies for such items as physicians' office space and major equipment. Moreover, these planning agencies are often dominated by local physicians hostile to HMOs. A 1973 study found that in states with certificate-of-need laws in effect or pending, 48% of the HMOs surveyed cited such laws as moderate or severe barriers to growth.[17]

Some states also impose "open enrollment" for HMOs but not for fee-for-service insurers. Open enrollment generally means that the insurer must accept all individuals, up to a certain number, in the order

[14]Richard McNeil and Robert Schlenker, "HMOs, Competition, and Government," *Health and Society*, Spring 1975, p. 198.

[15]Robert T. Holley and Rick J. Carlson, "The Legal Context for the Development of Health Maintenance Organizations," *Stanford Law Review* 24 (April 1972): 657.

[16]Frank Sloan and Roger Feldman, "Competition Among Physicians," in Warren Greenberg, ed., *Competition in the Health Care Sector: Past, Present and Future* (Germantown, Md.: Aspen Systems Corporation, 1978), p. 104.

[17]McNeil and Schlenker, p. 209.

in which they apply and without regard to their health status. Such requirements, therefore, prevent the insurer from discriminating among potential customers on the basis of perceived risk. One study found that an HMO's cost to persons joining during an open-enrollment period was 80% greater than it was for enrollees at other times.[18]

Advertising restrictions represent another potential threat to HMO development. The ability to advertise its services is critical to an HMO's survival because a large enrollment is necessary if the organization is to take full advantage of potential economies of scale. Yet because they provide medical services, HMOs are potentially subject to advertising restrictions that do no apply to fee-for-service insurers. For example, a Missouri law provides that the state may refuse to license a physician who engages in "unprofessional conduct." Included in the definition of "unprofessional conduct" is the solicitation of patients. In the case of an osteopath who was both chief of staff of and a shareholder in a clinic, a court held that the physician could not accomplish indirectly through the clinic what he could not do directly by himself.[19]

Recent Developments in Federal Law

The HMO Act of 1973 and the 1976 Amendments to the 1973 act are the basis of current federal policy toward HMOs. What these acts essentially do is override a number of state restrictions on HMOs that are actually or potentially federally certified. In particular, federal legislation overrides state legislation that (1) requires medical society approval and/or physician control; (2) imposes certain financial reserve requirements; and (3) forbids HMOs to advertise.

Federal legislation also provides for taxpayer subsidies to federally certified HMOs. For example, under interim regulations published in the *Federal Register* in March 1980, an HMO can receive up to $4 million in direct loans or in guaranteed loans to cover its start-up costs. In addition, certified HMOs can receive up to $2.5 million more in direct or guaranteed loans to construct or buy facilities.[20]

It is interesting that in making these subsidies available, the govern-

[18]Walter J. McClure, "Detrimental Effects of Applying the Present Medicare Amendments to Medicaid," Memo. (Minneapolis: Inter-Study, 1973). Cited in McNeil and Schlenker, p. 219.

[19]Holley and Carlson, p. 658.

[20]"U.S. Increases Money Available to Health Maintenance Systems," *New York Times*, 13 April 1980.

ment discriminates against for-profit HMOs. In general, for-profit HMOs can become federally certified along with nonprofit HMOs, but for-profit HMOs can qualify for federal loans and loan guarantees only if they meet a special requirement not imposed on nonprofit HMOs — at least 10% of the members projected to be served must be in an area that "lacks adequate medical facilities."[21]

Federally certified HMOs also enjoy another benefit denied fee-for-service insurers or noncertified HMOs. Federal law requires all employers with more than twenty-five employees who make a health benefits plan available to their employees to give their employees a dual option: If a federally certified HMO exists in the area, the employees must be given the option of receiving its services instead of fee-for-service insurance.

Although federal policy toward HMOs is widely interpreted as encouraging competition, it is not clear that free competition will be the ultimate result of the policy. Many health economists regard the amount of federal subsidy made available to HMOs as quite modest in the light of the disadvantages often imposed at the state and local levels, yet substantial subsidies coupled with the favoritism implicit in the "dual option" provision could lead to the creation of local monopolies.

A more serious problem, for the moment, is that once certified, HMOs are not given a free hand to compete with their rivals. Instead, they are saddled with a host of regulations.[22] Federally certified HMOs are required to offer a very generous package — more comprehensive than uncertified HMOs' benefits have traditionally been. For example, under federal law HMOs are required to offer short-term mental health services and alcoholism and drug-abuse services. They are also required to have open-enrollment periods during which they must accept all customers, regardless of health status.

In addition, HMOs are forbidden to vary the cost of their premiums to enrollees according to differences in perceived health risks. The same premium must be charged to all members of a given community. Federal law also requires an HMO to have one-third of its policy-making board made up of enrollees, limits HMOs from purchasing re-insurance, and imposes other reporting, quality-assurance, and continuing education requirements. There is also the unfortunate fact that once certified federal regulation becomes permanent; there is no mecha-

[21]Ibid.

[22]These regulations are summarized in McNeil and Schlenker, p. 216 f.

nism by which an HMO can become decertified and escape current and future regulatory restrictions.

The upshot is that federal law, although moving slightly in the direction of more competition, may simply be laying the groundwork for a federally regulated health care marketplace. As Clark Havighurst laments, "Under present conditions, the successful creation of an HMO is a triumph of managerial, legal, political, financial, marketing and negotiating skill. . . . The severe difficulties faced by HMOs, which Congress has done more to create than alleviate, make all the more important the encouragement of other private-sector efforts."[23]

[23]Clark C. Havighurst, "The Role of Competition in Cost Containment," p. 373–74.

VIII. MORE REGULATION

Entry can be barred by an obliging regulatory agency that equates public need to the private greed of the existing firms in the market.

Richard Posner
"Certificates of Need for Health Facilities:
A Dissenting View"

Although federal policy toward HMOs appeared to foster competition, the thrust of most new policy changes has been toward more centralization and control. In this chapter we shall look at some of the major types of regulation adopted in recent years: certificate-of-need laws, Professional Standards Review Organizations (PSROs), controls on hospital rates, budgets, and expenditures, and the Medical Device Amendments.

Before looking at these new regulatory devices, however, we need first to consider a problem cited as a reason for increased regulation of the medical marketplace: the problem of excess capacity.

The "Excess Capacity" Argument

The major reason given for most of the new regulatory mechanisms introduced in recent years is that there is an "excess capacity" in the hospital industry. That is, there are too many hospitals, too many beds, and too many pieces of modern medical equipment. This excess capacity is costly, and therefore, it is argued, it contributes to our rising national health care bill, often in the form of higher patient charges.

A recent report by the Institute of Medicine, for example, concluded that the United States has a significant surplus of hospital beds and recommended a reduction from the current stock of 4.4 beds per 1,000 persons to 4.0 per 1,000.[1] Studies of surgical and diagnostic facilities have also concluded that we have more of these facilities than we

[1]Institute of Medicine, *Controlling the Supply of Hospital Beds* (Washington, D.C.: National Academy of Sciences, 1976), pp. vii–ix and 7–16.

"need" — too many cardiac care units, too many radiation therapy installations, too may CAT scanners, etc.[2]

The excess capacity problem leads to a related problem: overutilization of medical facilities. Numerous studies have confirmed that additional hospital beds usually lead to additional hospital admissions and longer stays,[3] and that additional sophisticated equipment leads to more extensive use of complicated diagnostic and therapeutic medical procedures.[4] This greater utilization, of course, requires additional manpower and other support services and thus contributes in another way to rising medical costs.

Do we have more medical facilities than we really need? The term "need" is almost impossible to define and is rarely used by modern health economists. One reason is that there appears to be no limit to the amount of health care we can usefully consume. If there is such a limit, it definitely exceeds our annual gross national product.[5] A more meaningful question is this: Do we have more medical facilities than the public would want and be willing to pay for if they themselves bore the full cost of the medical services they consume? A tentative answer to this question is yes. As we saw in chapter 5, when the average hospital patient bears only 8 percent of his hospital bill in the form of out-of-pocket costs, he has an incentive to consume a great many medical services whose costs exceed the marginal value to the consumer. Under fee-for-service medical insurance, the providers of medical care have an incentive to oversupply services, and thus forces on both the demand and supply side of the market tend to push us

[2]For a recent summary of the case, see Walter McClure, *Reducing Excess Hospital Capacity* (Bureau of Health Planning and Resources Development, Department of Health, Education and Welfare, 1976), pp. 21–28. For an interesting but largely anecdotal description of the problem, see Judith Randal, "Wasteful Duplication in Our Hospitals," *The Reporter*, 15 December 1966, pp. 35–38.

[3]See Milton Roemer, "Bed Supply and Hospital Utilization: A Natural," *Hospitals, Journal of the American Hospital Association* 35 (November 1961): 36–42. The effect described is sometimes referred to as "Roemer's Law." See also Martin Feldstein, "Hospital Cost Inflation: A Study in Nonprofit Price Dynamics," *American Economic Review* 61 (December 1971): 853–72.

[4]Ralph Berry, "Cost and Efficiency in the Production of Hospital Services," *Milbank Memorial Fund Quarterly: Health and Society* 52 (Summer 1974): 291–313; and Karen Davis, "The Role of Technology, Demand and Labor Markets in the Determination of Hospital Cost," in Mark Perlman, ed., *The Economics of Health and Medical Care* (New York: Wiley, 1974), pp. 283–301.

[5]See John C. Goodman, *National Health Care in Great Britain: Lessons for the U.S.A.* (Dallas: Fisher Institute, 1980), chap. 4.

toward a greater utilization of medical facilities than would be the case if we bore the full cost of our actions at the time we took those actions.

Before we conclude that the problem is one requiring more government regulation of health facilities, however, we should remember that the "excess capacity" argument is a perennial cry of industries that seek protective regulations from the state. As Richard Posner has explained, "Every industry. . .believes that it has excess capacity, which is another way of saying it would like to reduce output and charge higher prices."[6] Indeed, the power of the state to eliminate excess capacity is the very same power that is often sought by industries in order to create an effective cartel for the purpose of maximizing industry profits. As Posner explains,

> Quite apart from any genuine danger of wasteful duplication of facilities, construction controls in regulated industries often serve to reinforce cartelization among the regulated firms. In the absence of such controls, members of the cartel would be tempted to cheat by expanding output beyond the quota fixed for each, and if any of them yielded to this temptation the cartel would eventually collapse. Control of construction can be used to limit expansion of output. If the cartel dominates the regulatory agency, as is unfortunately often the case, construction will not be permitted where the result would be overcapacity from the standpoint of maximizing cartel profits.[7]

Two interesting facts about the medical marketplace make Posner's warning especially forceful. First, although the health care industry is alleged to be characterized by excess capacity, this excess capacity does not seem to deter entry into the market. A great many newcomers apparently believe that the market offers them plenty of room to survive profitably. Second, the major regulatory mechanisms we shall look at in this chapter are not designed to close down existing facilities; all *are* designed to prevent the expansion of new ones.[8] As we shall see, this means that the regulatory structure is designed and functions to deter entry.

[6]Richard Posner, "Discussant's Comments," in Clark Havighurst, *Regulating Health Facilities Construction: Proceedings of a Conference on Health Planning, Certificates of Need, and Market Entry* (Washington, D.C.: American Enterprise Institute for Public Policy Research, 1974), p. 125.

[7]Richard Posner, "Certificates of Need for Health Facilities: A Dissenting View," in Havighurst, *Regulating Health Facilities Construction*, p. 114.

[8]No state certificate of need law, for example, gives regulatory bodies the power to close down beds; their only power is to limit expansion. See Clark Havighurst, "Regulation of Health Facilities and Services by Certificate of Need," *Virginia Law Review* 59 (October 1973): 1202.

Why should firms want to enter markets previously characterized by excess capacity? One explanation is that the hospital marketplace already functions as a quasi cartel. Moreover, it is a price-discriminating quasi cartel.[9] On the average, prices exceed true average costs, and prices on individual services do not reflect marginal production costs. It is precisely by such an environment that new entrants are attracted.[10] For example, if a service can be produced at a cost of $5 and patients charged a price of $10 for it, potential entrants will be tempted to enter the market and offer the same service for the slightly lower price of, say, $9.

This insight into the excess capacity problem explains why new entrants are attracted to the market. It also explains another important fact about the industry: Many of the major regulatory mechanisms we shall look at in this chapter came into existence with the active support of the groups who were to be regulated. Whether these groups will be able to control or "capture" the regulatory process and use it to promote their own interests remains to be seen.

Certificate-of-need Regulation

One of the most significant forms of regulation to develop in recent years is the certificate-of-need law. By 1973 twenty-three states had adopted such laws.[11] The National Health Planning and Resources Act of 1974 required all states to adopt certificate-of-need laws by 1980. The same act led to the establishment of about 200 Health Systems Agencies (HSAs), each governing a specific geographic area, to administer the certificate-of-need laws.

Generally speaking, certificate-of-need laws require hospitals to obtain approval from government planning agencies before they make major capital expenditures on physical plant, equipment, and services.[12] The size of expenditure requiring approval varies considerably from state to state, however. For example, in 1974 the dollar thresholds for spending on facilities ranged from $15,000 in Arizona to

9See David Salkever, "Competition Among Hospitals" in Warren Greenberg, ed., *Competition in the Health Care Sector: Past, Present and Future* (Germantown, Md.: Aspen Systems Corporation, 1978), pp. 191–206.

10Duncan Neuhauser, "The Future of Proprietaries in American Health Services," in Havighurst, *Regulating Health Facilities Construction*, p. 240.

11Clark C. Havighurst, "Regulation of Health Facilities and Services by 'Certificate of Need,'" *Virginia Law Review* 59, no. 7 (October 1973): 1144.

12Some states also require approval for the discontinuation of services and facilities.

$350,000 in Kansas; thresholds for spending on equipment ranged from $10,000 in Colorado to $100,000 in seven other states.[13]

The ostensible purpose of certificate-of-need legislation is to prevent overinvestment in facilities, equipment, and services and thereby hold down the cost of medical care. There has been no evidence that these programs have achieved this objective. One study, reviewing the record through 1974, concluded that "there is no evidence supporting the effectiveness or efficiency of capital expenditures regulation."[14] A more recent study by Salkever and Bice, found that certificate-of-need regulation resulted in no change in the amount of the investments by hospitals, although it did change the composition of those investments. The regulation resulted in less investment in beds and more investment in other kinds of hospital equipment. The study also indicates that certificate-of-need regulation may have increased overall hospital costs.[15]

The fact that certificate-of-need legislation has had little discernible effect on overall hospital investment does not mean that such regulation is not pernicious. In fact, a large number of health economists have warned that such regulation is likely to result in a de facto cartel operating in the interests of the hospitals.[16] The fact that the American Hospital Association has supported certificate-of-need laws since 1968 suggests that such a result is likely.[17] In addition, a number of state hospital associations have actively supported such legislation in several states.[18]

Certificate-of-need laws have also been supported by groups with a consumer's interest in hospital costs — for example, labor unions and

[13]David Salkever and Thomas Bice, *Hospital Certificate-of-Need Controls: Impact on Investment, Costs and Use* (Washington, D.C.: American Enterprise Institute for Public Policy Reseach, 1979), p. 6.

[14]Patrick O'Donoghue and Policy Center, Inc., *Evidence about the Effects of Health Care Regulation* (Denver: Spectrum Research, 1974), p. 67.

[15]Salkever and Bice, p. 75.

[16]See, for example, Clark C. Havighurst, "Regulation of Health Institutions," in Institute of Medicine, *Controls on Health Care* (Washington, D.C.: National Academy of Sciences, 1975), p. 81, and Richard Posner, "Certificates of Need for Health Facilities: A Dissenting View," p. 115.

[17]See William J. Curran, "A National Survey and Analysis of State Certificate-of-Need Laws for Health Facilities," in Clark C. Havighurst, *Regulating Health Facilities Construction*, p. 89.

[18]Macro Systems, Inc., *The Certificate of Need Experience: An Early Assessment* (Silver Spring, Md.: Macro Systems, 1974), vol. 2.

business groups,[19] and insurance interests, including Blue Cross–Blue Shield.[20] But if certificate-of-need regulation follows the trend established by regulation in other fields, it will be the providers, rather than consumers, who will have the upper hand with the planning agencies.[21]

In principle, the planning agencies have members representing consumer as well as producer interests, but a recent survey found that in most meetings devoted to certificate-of-need applications, the majority of members present were representatives of the providers of care.[22] In addition, these agencies often have a financial reason to favor the interests of the hospitals they regulate. With limited state and federal funding available, planning agencies often rely on contributions from local sources. Hospitals are major donors.[23]

The providers also have an advantage in terms of information and expertise. In theory, the planning agencies are supposed to determine the health "needs" of their regions and ensure that the facilities are available to meet those needs. In practice, decisions are apparently made on the basis of incomplete information. A General Accounting Office survey found that "less than half of the 163 health planning agencies . . . [surveyed] indicated knowledge of 1972 needs for types of inpatient and extended and ambulatory care facilities and beds. . . . The number knowing 1975 beds was even lower. . . . Most knew the number of existing health facilities."[24] A more recent survey of planning agencies in twenty states found the agencies relying extensively on information that was admittedly inadequate and obsolete.[25] In this context, the providers' access to pertinent information gives them a

19Curran, p. 89.

20Stuart Altman and Sanford Weiner, "Regulation as a Second Best," in Warren Greenberg, ed., *Competition in the Health Care Sector: Past, Present, and Future* (Germantown, Md.: Aspen Systems Corporation, 1978), p. 436.

21See Robert Helms, "The Health Cost Problem: Is Regulation Our Only Hope?" *Bulletin of the New York Academy of Medicine* 56, no. 1 (January-February 1980): 26–37.

22Lewin and Associates, Inc., *Evaluation of the Efficiency and Effectiveness of the Section 1122 Review Process* (Springfield, Va.: National Technical Information Service, 1975), part 1, pp. 1-16 - 1-17.

23Salkever and Bice, p. 16.

24Comptroller General of the United States, *Comprehensive Health Planning as Carried Out by States and Areawide Agencies in Three States* (Washington, D.C.: Government Printing Office, 1974), p. 18.

25Lewin and Associates, chap. 3.

distinct advantage over consumers in arguing their case before the planning agency.

Moreover, if conflicts develop between provider and consumer interests, the providers have a distinct edge in being able to take advantage of a preexisting organizational structure. As Salkever and Bice explain, the "providers have access to information, clinical assistance, and legal counsel from their respective institutions and trade associations that are unlikely to be equaled by resources available to consumers."[26]

The organizational disparity between the providers and the consumers is apparently even more important in bringing political pressure to bear on the planning agencies:

> Large, politically powerful institutions willing to devote considerable resources to defending their proposals through appeals, legal action, or legislative attempts to override agency decisions threaten to deplete agency resources and, if successful, to tarnish the agency's public image as a fair and effective regulatory body. This would suggest that certificate-of-need controls will be applied selectively among existing providers, favoring those with access to economic or political power.[27]

There is direct evidence to support this contention. Havighurst reports that planning agency files on applications frequently contain letters from legislators and public officials. Some applications were frankly described as "politically touchy." In one file, a memorandum discussed the political pressure being exerted by interested parties and made a judgment on the political wisdom of accepting the application.[28]

There is also direct evidence about the frequency with which certain types of applications are accepted or turned down. One study noted that there is a higher disapproval rate by planning agencies on applications submitted by proprietary than nonproprietary institutions.[29] Other studies have noted that HMOs are frequently disadvantaged in planning agency decisions.[30]

[26]Salkever and Bice, p. 16. See also William J. Bicknell and Diana C. Walsh, "Critical Experiences in Organizing and Administrating a State Certificate-of-Need Program," *Public Health Reports* 91 (January-February 1976), pp. 29–45.

[27]Salkever and Bice, pp. 18–19.

[28]Havighurst, "Regulation of Health Facilities and Services," p. 1186, n. 158.

[29]Lewin and Associates, pp. 5-19 – 5-22.

[30]Havighurst, "Regulation of Health Facilities and Services," pp. 1208 f.

Havighurst has described the trend toward cartelization:

> Limited investigation suggests . . . that established community hospitals, major medical centers, hospitals associated with religious and similar organizations, and well-entrenched proprietaries seem to be capable of receiving special attention for applications which would be rejected out of hand if submitted by less well-connected interests. The long-run consequence of such systematic preferences is that larger hospitals grow while new facilities are discouraged; incumbents enjoy an unwritten presumption in proposing to replace their outmoded facilities; "satellites" of existing hospitals are favored over new entrants; and "chains" and other proprietaries are excluded in favor of existing facilities or community-sponsored organizations. Perhaps economics of scale and quality considerations could in some measure justify these tendencies, but the end result is less consumer choice and more concentrated control in local markets.[31]

PSROs

Professional Standards Review Organizations (PSROs) were mandated at the national level under provisions of the Social Security Amendments Act of 1972.[32] According to the legislation, panels of local physicians are to monitor care provided to Medicare and Medicaid patients by hospitals, extended care facilities, and skilled nursing homes. The law requires PSROs to determine whether the care provided is (or was) (1) medically necessary, (2) of professional quality, and (3) delivered in an appropriate health care facility, e.g., on an inpatient basis only when outpatient care is inappropriate.

Although the law provides for some overall national supervision through a National Professional Standards Review Council, each PSRO is encouraged to establish its own norms for diagnosis and treatment based on the perceived patterns of practice in its own geographic area. Prior to 1 January 1976 physicians were encouraged to voluntarily form PSROs in their localities and receive federal funds for the operation of these organizations once they had been recognized by the Secretary of Health, Education and Welfare. If more than 10 percent of the physicians in an area objected to a PSRO on the grounds that it was unrepresentative of area physicians, HEW was obliged to poll local physicians. If more than half the physicians in an area voted against the PSRO, it could not be designated. After 1 January 1976

[31]Ibid., pp. 1186–87.

[32]For an analysis of the legal background for the establishment of PSROs, see Cedric Chao, "Cost and Quality Control in the Medicare/Medicaid Program: Concurrent Review," *Harvard Civil Rights – Civil Liberties Law Review* 11 (1976): 664–700.

HEW was given the authority to designate PSROs in areas where they had not been voluntarily established.

Physicians are encouraged to comply with PSRO decisions in three principal ways. First, PSROs have direct authority to deny approval of payment for services to physicians who provide care to Medicare and Medicaid patients. Second, the law includes a malpractice exemption for physicians who conform with or rely on PSRO norms, provided that they exercise due care during the course of treatment. Finally, PSROs have the power to impose specific sanctions on physicians who do not meet "professionally recognized standards," and, ultimately, to exclude such physicians from reimbursement under Medicaid-Medicare programs. PSROs even have the authority to fine individual physicians.[33]

Ostensibly, PSRO regulation pertains only to medical care administered under certain government programs, but in practice the decisions of PSROs are potentially much more far-reaching. For one thing, by prior agreement with PSROs, private insurers may have PSROs review the cases of patients with private health insurance.[34] For another, political pressure is developing to extend PSRO reviews to all patients, whether or not they are covered by federal programs.[35] But the most important effect of PSRO standards is the implication for malpractice law.

Since the 1972 Social Security Amendments Act attempts to shield physicians who treat Medicare and Medicaid patients from malpractice liability if they observe PSRO standards, it is likely that physicians treating other patients will be encouraged to follow those same norms, especially if the courts treat PSRO norms as judicial norms in adjudicating malpractice cases. For example, once a PSRO establishes a minimum length of hospitalization for a certain treatment in its area, it is highly likely that all physicians and institutions in the area will adhere to this minimum standard.[36]

PSROs are widely regarded as a regulatory mechanism for reducing

[33]See Frank Sloan and Roger Feldman, "Competition Among Physicians," in Greenberg, ed., *Competition in the Health Care Sector*, p. 106.

[34]Clark C. Havighurst and Randall Bovbjerg, "Professional Standards Review Organizations and Health Maintenance Organizations: Are They Compatible?" *Utah Law Review* 381 (Summer 1975): 391.

[35]Ibid., pp. 391–92, n. 44. See also, Council on Wage and Price Stability, *The Complex Puzzle of Rising Health Care Costs: Can The Private Sector Fit It Together?* (Washington, D.C.: Government Printing Office, 1976), p. 27.

[36]Havighurst and Bovbjerg, p. 395.

the costs of health care. Indeed, two of the stated aims of PSRO reviews are directly related to health care costs — the aim of eliminating unnecessary medical treatment and the aim of eliminating unnecessary institutionalization of patients. Yet there is no evidence that PSROs have succeeded in achieving these aims. In fact, an HEW evaluation of the PSRO program found that by the end of 1976 the costs of the program exceeded its benefits. The HEW report concluded that the "data are sufficient to strongly suggest that PSRO implementation alone is not apt to cause significant changes in either hospitalization rates or associated government expenditures."[37]

That PSROs have not achieved their aims is hardly surprising. In the first place, PSROs, controlled by panels of local physicians, have no incentive to achieve them. As Sloan and Feldman ask, "Why should a board of practicing physicians curb utilization and hence Federal payments to its locality?"[38] In the second place, the norms established by PSROs are likely to be derived from an average based on the locality's previous experiences. Physicians and institutions who were previously above the average will be encouraged to move toward it, and so will those who were previously below it. PSROs are likely to create uniformity, but there is no obvious reason why the established norms should be substantially different from the pre-PSRO average experience of the locality.

In the third place, there is a direct conflict between the cost-reducing aims of the program and its third objective: maintaining professional quality. Higher quality medical care, as we have seen, is almost always more expensive medical care.[39] The potential conflict between the quality-enhancing and cost-reducing features of the program was recognized by government officials from the outset. In fact, in attempting to sell the PSRO program to the medical community, HEW expressly

[37]U.S. Department of Health, Education and Welfare, *PSRO: An Evaluation of the Professional Standards Review Organization, Executive Summary,* draft (Washington, D.C., 1977), pp. i–iv; cited in American Enterprise Institute, *Proposals for the Regulation of Hospital Costs* (Washington, D.C.: American Enterprise Institute for Public Policy Research, 1978), p. 13.

[38]Sloan and Feldman, p. 108.

[39]For a discussion of quality-cost tradeoffs, see Clark C. Havighurst and James F. Blumstein, "Coping with Quality/Cost Tradeoffs in Medical Care: The Role of PSROs," *Northwestern University Law Review* 70, no. 6 (March-April 1975): 6–68; and James F. Blumstein, "Inflation and Quality: The Case of the PSROs," in M. Zubkoff, ed., *Health: A Victim or a Cause of Inflation* (New York: Milbank Memorial Fund, 1976), pp. 245–95.

declared that the law's primary purpose was to assure quality.[40]

That the PSRO program can be used as a vehicle to enchance the quality of medical care is perhaps its most significant feature. As we have seen in previous chapters, organized medicine has often used the publicly-stated goal of "quality" as a pretense for eliminating competition and raising the incomes of the providers of medical care. Potentially, PSROs could be used in a like manner. Indeed, as early as 1974 Clark Havighurst warned that PSROs could foster cartellike regulation.[41]

That the AMA has publicly opposed the PSRO program does not mean that organized medicine is unwilling to use the program to pursue its traditional objectives.[42] For example, the director of the AMA's Center for Health Services Research and Development has said of PSROs:

> It seems apparent after examining the legislation that the primary, if not total intent of the program is to contain the *cost* of medical care.
>
> Despite the legislative intent of the program, however, the concern of health care providers and insurers should be to reassign priorities of the PSRO program to assure that maintenance of high quality care is the *primary* focus of PSROs.[43]

The PSRO program could be used to further the cartel objectives of medical providers in a manner similar to the ways in which other quality control techniques have been used in the past. Take length of stay for certain treatments, for example. As we have seen, proprietary hospitals tend to have shorter lengths of stay than conventional voluntary hospitals for the same treatment. PSROs are certain to be dominated by physicians and hospitals who see the proprietaries as a threat, and, as a consequence, the PSRO might establish a normative minimum length of stay that reflects the experience of voluntary hospitals. If the proprietaries failed to meet these standards they would be jeop-

[40]In an explanatory pamphlet, expressly aimed at physicians, HEW asked itself the question, "Is the purpose of PSRO to assure quality or cost control?" and answered, "The primary emphasis of the PSRO program is on assuring the quality of medical care." See *PSRO: Questions and Answers* (Washington, D.C.: HEW, 1973); cited in Havighurst and Bovbjerg, pp. 390–91, n. 38.

[41]Havighurst, "Regulation of Health Institutions," p. 81.

[42]"The Complex Puzzle of Rising Health Care Costs," p. 27.

[43]"Towards a Strategy for Evaluating PSROs," *Westchester Medical Bulletin*, November 1974. Cited in Clark C. Havighurst, "Federal Regulation of the Health Care Delivery System: A Foreword in the Nature of a 'Package Insert,'" *Toledo Law Review* 6 (Spring 1975): 581, n. 9.

ardized by the penalties the PSROs are empowered to inflict. If they did meet the PSRO standards, however, the proprietary hospitals would lose the competitive advantage they bring to the marketplace.

Similar concerns apply to any institution that tries to practice medicine innovatively and compete vigorously for patients. For example, Havighurst and Bovbjerg have stressed that

> there are serious hazards in exposing [HMOs] to possible domination by fee-for-service practitioners through the PSRO mechanism. Preservation of the HMOs capacity to allocate resources to their best uses and to conserve resources by substituting inputs and omitting expensive steps contributing little or nothing to better outcomes is essential to its success from any point of view.... The result could well be the elimination of many of those very features which distinguish the HMO from fee-for-service medicine and make it an attractive mechanism for expanding the range of services available to many populations.[44]

Other Forms of Regulation

In the light of so much recent criticism of the nation's health care system and of a plethora of regulatory proposals currently pending before Congress, most Americans would probably be surprised to learn how much regulation already exists. Roughly one-third of the nation's community hospitals now have their rates, revenues, or budgets regulated at the state level.[45] In addition there are a host of other state, local, and federal regulations ranging from the licensing of hospital personnel to government-mandated fire, safety, and building codes.

Just how extensive government regulations are recently came to light during testimony before the Council on Wage and Price Stability: A hospital in New York is now governed by 99 separate regulatory agencies; a hospital in New Jersey is governed by 119 regulatory bodies; over 500 government regulations apply to nursing homes. A pathologist in Florida complained of "thirty-odd governmental regulatory agencies that regulate or are looking over my shoulder."[46]

Although many of these regulations were designed to keep health care costs down, the cost of complying with regulations can itself be quite high. Consider the cost of paperwork: A hospital administrator in Ohio reported that in order to satisfy a requirement mandating the

[44]Havighurst and Bovbjerg, pp. 388–89.

[45]Congressional Budget Office, *Controlling Rising Hospital Costs* (Washington, D.C.: Government Printing Office, 1979), p. 55.

[46]"The Complex Puzzle of Rising Health Care Costs," p. 14.

use of one reporting form, an $8,000 employee had to be hired. If each of the nations 7,000 hospitals had a similar experience, national health expenditures would rise by $56 million.[47] A member of the National Council of Health Care Services estimated the cost of preparing Medicare and Medicaid reports at $1,000 per facility per report. If each of the 12,000 nursing homes that participate in Medicare and Medicaid prepare 1.86 reports per year, the annual cost of paper work is $22,320,000.[48]

It is not known what overall effects have been produced by the complex regulatory net that has fallen over the health care industry. However, a recent study of 1,228 hospitals focused on some of the major forms of regulation, including certificate-of-need regulation, PSRO regulation, and hospital revenue controls. The study found that new, comprehensive regulatory programs had no effect on hospital costs. It found that more mature, noncomprehensive programs increased total expenses per patient per day by almost 5 percent in the short run and by almost 10 percent in the long run.[49]

Professor George Hilton has described regulatory commissions as having a tendency "to generate monopoly gain in one activity, either through administering a cartel or maintaining a monopoly, and then to dissipate it in uneconomic activity."[50] It appears from the recent trends that regulation of the health care industry will prove to be no exception to the general rule.

The Medical Device Amendments

One of the most revolutionary events in modern medicine has been the development and use of artificial organs and biomedical devices. Today, artificial medical devices are used in virtually every area of medicine. Some of the more exotic of these devices are the artificial kidney and the artificial heart, but there are also heart valves, pacemakers, heart-lung machines, artificial elbows, knees, hips, and computerized eyes. So rapid has been the development of medical devices

[47] Ibid., p. 15.

[48] Ibid., p. 17.

[49] F. A. Sloan and B. Steinwald, "Effects of Regulation on Hospital Costs and Input Use." (Paper presented to the Annual Meeting of the American Economic Association, Chicago, 29 August 1978).

[50] George Hilton, "The Basic Behavior of Regulatory Commissions," *American Economic Review* 62, no. 47 (1972): 50.

that in 1976 over $45 million was spent in the United States on plastic biomedical devices.[51]

That same year an important political event took place that threatens the future development of new medical devices and promises to increase their cost greatly. This was the passage of the Medical Device Amendments to the Food, Drug and Cosmetic Act. These amendments gave additional powers to the Food and Drug Administration (FDA) to regulate medical devices.

Prior to 1976 the FDA could act to remove a medical device from the market only if the device was shown to be harmful. This standard was quite different from the standard applied to new drugs. Under the 1962 amendments to the Food, Drug and Cosmetic Act, new drugs had to be tested and shown to be safe and effective *before* they were allowed on the market. After July 1980, when the Medical Device Amendments became effective, however, some of the same standards that applied to drugs were applied to medical devices. Under current law medical devices must be tested and must win FDA approval before they can be marketed. The exact procedures differ according to the estimated "degree of risk" associated with the device.

Why are the Medical Device Amendments so important? Consider our experience with FDA regulation of new drugs. Over the past two decades, the process by which a new drug receives approval from the FDA has become increasingly complicated, lengthy, and costly. A little over fifteen years ago it took an average of about two years from the time that drug evaluation was begun in human beings to the time the drug was approved for marketing. Today that process takes almost nine years.[52] It has been estimated that the FDA reviews an average of 120,000 pages of complex data for each drug. The research costs to the pharmaceutical firms of preparing such reports have increased enormously. In 1962 R & D cost per new chemical entity was estimated to be about $4 million. Today that figure is over $50 million.[53] The increased delays and increased costs of the approval pro-

51L. Craig Metcalf, "Legal Problems in Medical Device Development," *Insurance Council Journal*, July 1977, p. 408.

52Center for the Study of Drug Development, University of Rochester, "Preliminary Analyses of 1977 U.S. Investigational New Chemical Entity (NCE) Study," mimeographed, p. 2; cited in Gerald Laubach, "Federal Regulation and Pharmaceutical Innovation," in Arthur Levin, ed., *Regulating Health Care: The Struggle for Control* (*Proceedings of the Academy of Political Science* 33, no. 4 (1980), p. 63).

53Ronald W. Hansen, "The Pharmaceutical Development Process: Estimates of Development Costs and Times and the Effects of Proposed Regulatory Changes," in

cess have had a pronounced effect: The number of new chemical entities introduced in the United States each year has declined from an average of fifty-two twenty years ago to sixteen in 1977 and twenty-three in 1978.[54]

One way of appreciating the harshness of the FDA approval process is to compare the experience of the United States with that of European countries. A recent study by the General Accounting Office found that thirteen out of fourteen especially important drugs approved by the FDA between July 1975 and February 1978 were available in other countries first — between two months and twelve years earlier than in the United States.[55] Another study comparing Britain and the United States found that from January 1977 to March 1979 four times as many new drugs became available in Britain as became available only in the United States.[56]

It is the almost unanimous opinion of health economists who have examined FDA policies that regulation of new drugs in recent years has been harmful to the public. Space does not permit a full discussion of the extent of this harm, but one class of drugs is especially noteworthy, the beta-blockers. These drugs are useful in treating hypertension and many of the symptoms of heart disease, including angina pectoris. They are also useful in cases of hard-to-treat cardiovascular disease. Yet despite these facts, a dozen or more beta-blockers that have been used for years in Europe are still unavailable in the United States. Professor William Wardell recently estimated that as many as 10,000 heart-related deaths per year might be prevented if the appropriate beta-blockers were available and in widespread use in this country.[57]

Robert L. Chien, ed., *Issues in Pharmaceutical Economics* (Lexington, Mass.: D. C. Heath and Company, 1979), p. 180.

[54]Laubach, pp. 62–63.

[55]"Statement of Gregory J. Ahart, Director, Human Resources Division (U.S. General Accounting Office) before the (U.S. House of Representatives) Committee on Science and Technology, Subcommittee on Science, Research and Technology, on the Food and Drug Administration's Drug Approval Process, June 19, 1979," mimeographed, p. 3.; cited in Laubach, p. 70.

[56]"Statement of William Wardell, M.D., Ph.D., at Hearings on the Food and Drug Administration's New Drug Approval Process, Submitted to the Science, Research and Technology Subcommittee of the Committee on Science and Technology, United States House of Representatives, June 19, 1979," mimeographed, pp. 3–7; cited in Laubach, p. 71.

[57]Ibid.

A complete analysis of FDA policies toward drugs lies beyond the scope of this book, but we have seen sufficient evidence of how the agency has traditionally treated innovation to be able to guess how it is likely to treat medical devices.

What would have happened had the current demand for medical devices been in effect a decade or so ago? Dr. Arthur Beall, the Baylor College of Medicine professor who invented an artificial heart valve in the 1960s, has noted that if heart valves were developed under the regulations in effect now, they would still not be commercially available. Dr. Belding Scribner, the University of Washington physician who helped develop renal dialysis for kidney patients, points to a similar problem in his field. Dr. Scribner's most recent innovation was the arteriovenus shunt, a man-made blood vessel (fashioned of Teflon) implanted in the arm to allow kidney patients to undergo repeated dialysis. Under the current regulations, he says, his group would undoubtedly have been forced to experiment first with dogs, yet these experiments would have failed because dog blood, as was shown later, coagulates exceptionally easily.[58]

Not all producers of medical devices were opposed to the recent changes in federal regulatory procedures. In fact, many of the large producers of medical devices have volunteered to aid the FDA in creating minimum standards for their products.[59] Small firms are in a different position, however. As in the case of the costly and prolonged approval process for new drugs, it will be the small manufacturing firms that will find it the most difficult to compete successfully. That eventuality will harm consumers in yet another way: Industry executives frankly admit that the smaller companies are often the most creative.[60]

[58]Sandy Graham, "Doctors, Firms Say New Rules Kill Creativity," *Wall Street Journal*, 28 July 1980, p. 13.

[59]Metcalf, p. 410.

[60]Graham, p. 13.

IX. CONCLUSION

Some form of national health insurance is exactly what we're heading into. What can we, as physicians, do in the face of the inevitable? We'd best concentrate our efforts, I think, not in opposing the concept but in devising the kind of program we can live with comfortably. It would have to be one that's good for our patients, of course — but it's up to us to make sure it's reasonable and fair to us.

Dr. John Fisher
Medical Economics, 1978

As the United States enters the 1980s, the prospects for a free market for medical care seem bleak. Congress has been flooded with proposals to establish a system of national health insurance with controls on health care spending placed firmly in the hands of federal regulators.

What can the public look forward to if such a system is adopted? One thing they should not expect is a more efficient health care system. With all of its inefficiencies, distorted incentives, and regulatory burdens, our health care system is still more efficient than the systems of countries with comprehensive national health insurance schemes. In fact, measured in terms of average-length-of-stay statistics, the United States has the most efficient health care system in the industrialized world.[1]

The evidence, then, suggests that comprehensive regulation will raise, not lower, the true cost of medical care. It also suggests that patients can look forward to a lower quality of care in return for the health care dollars spent. I recently compared some indicators of the quality of health care received by patients in five countries: the United States, Canada, West Germany, Norway, and Denmark.[2] In 1976 these countries spent similar amounts per capita on health care,

[1]See *Public Expenditures on Health*, The Organization for Economic Cooperation and Development (Paris: OECD, 1977), p. 19, table 5.

[2]John C. Goodman, "The Politics of Medicine," *Policy Review*, forthcoming.

although they had very different health care systems. The fraction of health care spending done by the United States government that year was approximately one-half what it was in the other four countries.

This difference between the role of government involvement in health care in the United States and in the other four countries appears to have led to important differences in the quality of health care. Although the amount spent on health care was similar in all five countries, the four countries with national health care systems devoted fewer resources to those types of care that are known to result in actual improvements in the health care of patients: The other four countries had fewer CAT scanners per capita, fewer dialysis machines per capita, and trained a much lower percentage of their physicians in specialized fields. Comparisons of mortality rates in these countries with those in the United States revealed that these differences in spending priorities affect the health of patients: For diseases for which medical intervention is known to make a real difference and for which lifestyle and environment are inconsequential causes of disease, the United States had significantly lower mortality rates.

Space does not permit an analysis of why government health care systems produce greater inefficiency and a lower quality of care than Americans receive under our current system. I have elaborated on the reasons for these phenomena elsewhere.[3] Suffice it to say that in the area of health care, as in so many other areas, the political marketplace operates differently from the economic marketplace.

Perhaps the most disturbing recent trend in health care politics is the attitude of so many of the providers of health care services. Although organized medicine and its allies in the health insurance, medical manufacturing, and pharmaceutical industries have so far resisted the more extreme proposals for comprehensive national health insurance, there is no assurance that they will continue to do so.

As the epigraph to this chapter indicates, many within the health care industry want to shape and mold national health insurance proposals to fit their own economic interests rather than oppose them outright. As they have in so many other countries, the producers of health care may soon become the architects of national health insurance in the United States.

The unfortunate result is that the burden of protecting our health

[3]John C. Goodman, *National Health Care in Great Britain: Lessons for the U.S.A.* (Dallas: The Fisher Institute, 1980), chap. 10.

care system from further government intrusions will probably fall squarely on the shoulders of the general public. My prediction is that if socialized medicine is ultimately defeated in this country, it will be patients, not doctors, who will be primarily responsible.

ABOUT THE AUTHOR

Dr. John C. Goodman is assistant professor of economics and Director of the Center for Health Policy Research at the University of Dallas.

Dr. Goodman received his Ph.D. in economics from Columbia University and has been engaged in teaching and research at over six colleges and universities, including Stanford University, Dartmouth College, and Sarah Lawrence College.

He is the author of *Economics of Public Policy: The Micro View* (with Edwin Dolan); *Opting Out of Social Security in Great Britain; National Health Care in Great Britain: Lessons for the U.S.A.*, and numerous articles in professional journals.